Hello HEALTHY

*Strategies to Reach Your Full
Health and Wellness Potential*

DR. WES YOUNGBERG

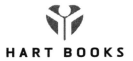

HART BOOKS

PO Box 2377, Fallbrook, CA 92088 · (800) 487-4278

Editor: Russell Holt
Design: Mark Bond for BONDesign
Typeset: 11 / 15 Dante

PRINTED IN U.S.A.

1 2 3 4 5 6 7 8 9 10

Youngberg, Wes
    Hello Healthy: Twelve Weeks to Wellness / Wes Youngberg–1st ed.
    Includes bibliographical references.
    ISBN: 978-1-878046-75-8
    1. Health—Health Concerns   2. Health—Disease   3. Health—Natural Cures

Also by Dr. Wes Youngberg: *Goodbye Diabetes*

To order additional copies of *Hello Healthy* by Dr. Wes Youngberg,
call 1-800-487-4278 or visit www.goodbyediabetes.com.

CONTENTS

FOREWORD V

1. ARE THERE HOLES IN YOUR GENES? *Reaching Your Full Genetic Potential* . . . 1

2. CALORIES IN, CALORIES OUT: *The Importance of Diet and Exercise* 16

3. MATTERS OF THE HEART: *Optimizing Circulation and Heart Health* 30

4. HERE COMES THE SUN! *Sunlight, Vitamin D and Health* 52

5. IT'S A GUT FEELING: *Optimizing Digestion* 74

6. STRESSED OUT: *Stress, Emotions and Adrenal Fatigue* 97

7. POSITIVELY HEALTHY: *Attitudes and Healing* 119

8. THE NEW NORMAL: *Chronic Kidney Disease* 138

9. FRIENDLY FIRE: *The Autoimmune Epidemic* 163

10. PLAYING WITH POISON: *Detoxification for Optimal Health* 188

11. REST IS BEST: *How Sleep Impacts Your Health* 221

12. TESTING... TESTING... *Choosing the Best Clinical Lab Tests* 242

APPENDIX 287

PLEASE NOTE: *This book contains stories and case studies involving patients the author has worked with in the past. Their names and identities have been changed to protect their privacy and in the interest of confidentiality. The information in this book is for educational purposes only. It is designed to help you make informed decisions about your health, but is not intended to be a substitute for professional medical advice. Always consult your healthcare provider to determine the appropriateness of the information for your own situation. If you need specific advice, seek help from a medical professional who is knowledgeable in that area. The author and publisher specifically disclaim all responsibility for any liability, loss, or risk, personal or otherwise, which is incurred as a consequence, directly or indirectly, of the use and application of any of the contents of this book.*

As I work with clients in my office, by phone, or by Skype, and as I speak at health seminars or medical conferences, people often ask, "Of all the health strategies we've been discussing and learning about—which is the most important?"

I usually smile and answer, "The most important health strategy for you is the one you're not following!"

If you're neglecting or overlooking a particular strategy for optimizing your health, you're not only depriving yourself of the benefits of that particular strategy, but you're also not taking advantage of the synergy that comes from the interaction between all the components of a comprehensive wellness program. Every time you add one more effective approach to the list of wellness strategies you're implementing, you get an exponential increase in your healing potential because of the synergy effect.

Hello Healthy is a book about helping you get this synergy effect by applying all the strategies necessary to reach your full health and wellness potential. The twelve chapters of this book are a series of twelve sessions in a practical program that you can follow as you go about your daily routine. These are twelve major strategies that I specifically address with each patient, regardless of their health concerns or wellness goals. They provide the foundation that each of us can use to master our genetic risk by actually turning off disease-causing genes and turning on the genes that promote health.

As you come to better understand the principles we'll be discussing—and incorporate them as part of your new lifestyle—you'll be able to enjoy a higher level of health and wellness than you've ever thought possible.

Hello Healthy is how friends and family may soon be addressing you!

— Wes Youngberg, DrPH, MPH, CNS, FACLM
Lifestyle Medicine Specialist & Clinical Nutritionist

ONE

Are There Holes in Your Genes?

REACHING YOUR FULL GENETIC POTENTIAL

DAVID'S WHOLE BODY WAS SHAKING. HIS BEAUTIFUL 5-year old daughter thought he was going to die. Could he turn this around—change the expression of his genes and reach his lifetime goals, including running the Honolulu marathon? How could this happen? Sudden questions, in need of urgent answers. Answers that require an understanding of something called the human genome.

THE HUMAN GENOME

The human genome is the sum total of all the genetic information in your body. Inside the nuclei of nearly every cell in your body are forty-six chromosomes. Half come from your father; half are from your mother. Your genetic blueprint is stored inside your genes on these chromosomes. The genes contain a code for making everything your body needs, especially proteins. Proteins are basic to life; they help carry out almost all the functions of the human body.

You have approximately 20,000 genes. The Human Genome Project successfully finished decoding and mapping these 20,000 genes in the spring of 2003. Scientists now knew the code and the structure of each human gene. This opened up vast new areas of genomic research—identifying which genes contribute to specific disease and developing new therapies to address genetic flaws.

EPIGENETICS

Most people believe that their medical destiny is determined by the genes they have inherited. In other words, each of us is dealt a certain genetic hand at birth, and the genes we have been given largely determine whether or not we will develop specific diseases or medical problems. According to this view, some people inherit "good" genes, and some people inherit "bad" genes. We don't have a choice; we must simply hope for the best. That has been the conventional wisdom regarding genetic theory for decades. However, recent research in the area of epigenetics has proven that this idea is not true. What is epigenetics?

The term, epigenetics comes from combining the Greek word, *epi*, meaning "in addition to" or "on top of," with the word *genetics*. So "epigenetics" refers to all the factors that affect the way genes work, independently of the genes themselves. One's epigenome, then, is made up of all the chemical compounds that have been added to the entirety of one's DNA (genome) as a way to regulate the activity of all the genes within the genome. Epigenetic changes can help determine whether genes are turned on or off and can influence the production of proteins in certain cells.

> No matter what genes we have, their expression and actions are influenced by thousands of different factors. The environment in which we live, the choices we make, and the habits we form all greatly affect how our genes function.

FAT YELLOW MICE

Some years ago I came across a study reported in a cellular biology journal that changed our entire perspective about what genetic risk really is. The study,[1] conducted by Dr. Randy Jirtle at the Duke University Genome Institute, involved agouti mice. Most mice are supposed to be lean, brown, and have a lot of energy. Agouti mice have been specially bred to be fat with yellow coats. They easily become diabetic or develop heart disease. Many of them die prematurely of cancer. That's a big triple, or quadruple, whammy!

The study divided these fat, yellow mice equally into two random groups. Each group received the same standard mouse diet, but one group also received some "super" nutrients, such as genistein found in whole soybeans and folate.

Folate, we now know, has such a powerful influence that it can actually bypass genetic mutations. That's right, you can literally bypass a major genetic mutation just by having enough of the right nutrient! Eating what I call "first-class foods" can powerfully alter your genetic risk for certain diseases and medical problems.

In the Duke University study, within a generation after these fat, yellow female mice began eating the right super nutrients, they started giving birth—not to fat, yellow mice—but to lean, brown-coated mice! The fat, yellow mothers and their lean, brown offspring had the same genes that coded for a dominant yellow coat and a predisposition to all those disease processes. So what happened? What accounted for the change? Although the lean, brown offspring had the same genetic makeup as their mothers, those genes coding for yellow coats and a predisposition to disease had been turned off! They were still there, but they had been deactivated.

The point is that all of us have genes in our bodies that could kill us if they were turned on. We also have genes in our body that, if turned on, could dramatically speed the healing potential that we all possess. It's all about finding a strategy, or a group of strategies, which can help us genetically activate and promote the healing process, while also slowing down the aging process. Of course, we're all going to get old. But my goal is to get old like Julie Phillips of Raynham, Massachusetts, who parachuted out of an airplane at the age of 90!

GENETIC CHANGE IS POSSIBLE

Given the right nutrients, these fat, unhealthy, yellow mice were able to give birth to mice that were healthy even though they inherited their mothers' unhealthy genes. That is an extremely important fact which applies not only to mice; it applies to you and me. That means that if you are a young person who plans to have children, you will not only transfer your genes to them, you'll also determine whether those genes are turned on or off in your children. This is an opportunity for you to make good choices now. Don't wait until you're in your 50s to say, "Maybe I should start taking care of my health." Start now! Your children will thank you their entire lives. You can dramatically transform the genetic expression of your children by paying attention to health habits in your own life now. That can be a sobering thought, but it can also be a very encouraging thought.

We can see this principle in action by examining identical twins. Take two identical twin girls at age 10. It's difficult to tell one from the other. Now fast forward fifty or sixty years. You clearly still have identical twins, but there are major differences between them. One is enjoying good health; the other has been diagnosed with terminal cancer. In such cases, we can't blame genetics. Obviously, something else has made the difference. That something is what epigenetics is all about—the study of all the environmental factors and all the lifestyle choices that have affected one's personal genetic expression.

> Today, we can analyze a sample of blood, saliva, or hair and match it to a genetic databank and determine to whom it belongs. That's a useful crime tool. But did you know that we can also analyze whether specific genes in a sample have been turned on or off?

That's a physiological test that can actually be done in the lab. This gives us the opportunity to study how a comprehensive lifestyle program can actually change a person's epigenome. This is a fascinating field and one that I'm excited to be involved with.

HOW IMPORTANT IS FAMILY HISTORY?

Often, when a person is confronted with a certain medical condition—heart disease or diabetes, for example—he or she will blame family history. There's an interesting study, the Archimedes Study, conducted by Dr. David Eddy,[2] that helps us put "family history" into its proper perspective. Dr. Eddy is a physician and well-known researcher who also has a Ph.D. in mathematics. He selected 10,000 individuals from National Institutes of Health studies and put all their health data into a computerized aging simulation, starting at age 20 and ending the study at age 80. The study controlled for various risk factors, but then "fixed" these risk factors one at a time in order to identify those factors that had the greatest impact on the health of the individuals being studied.

Do you know what this study found to be the least important of all those risk factors in terms of actually affecting the health outcome? Family history. When properly controlled for in this virtual simulated study, family history accounted for only 4 percent of the total risk of having a heart attack.

Now, that doesn't mean family history isn't important. After all, if you miss 4 percent of the questions in a test, you'd have to score essentially perfect on every other part of the test to get a top grade. So I'm not suggesting you pay no attention to your family history when looking at medical issues. Family history can help you focus on the right strategies for reaching your full genetic potential. Knowledge is power, and awareness of your personal risk for particular medical problems can motivate you to initiate transformational changes in your lifestyle. But family history isn't the most important genetic factor in determining your level of health.

Recent findings in genetic research are indicating that you can master your genetic risk with lifestyle and nutritional strategies.

That's important. Why? Because there is a lot of hopelessness in the world we live in today. Many people ask, "Why should I try to improve my health if it's all predetermined genetically at conception?" So we give up emotionally.

But the good news is that your genes have not set your health and wellness levels in stone. The good news is that change is possible! One of the most important things that I want you to take from this book is a sense of hope—a sense that transformational change is possible. And the second important concept I want to get across is that you can do it! You can reach your full genetic potential if you're willing to do what it takes and put some effort into the process. High blood pressure, diabetes, depression, chronic fatigue, joint pain—whatever ails you, whatever challenges you have, whatever your family history has placed in your family tree—there is hope for you!

IT'S NEVER TOO LATE

I see many middle-aged persons or elderly persons who finally realize that they need to do something about their health. (It's never too late, by the way, to begin making changes to transform your health.) But what really concerns me is that I'm seeing more and more patients in their late 20s and 30s. They have young children, and they are already suffering the consequences of chronic disease. They're already struggling with a high risk of liver failure, of kidney failure, heart disease, or diabetes. What about them? Is there any hope for them? Yes. Absolutely. Even those who are dealing with these kinds of issues at a young age can benefit from stepping back to look at the bigger perspective of health and lifestyle—and begin making those transformational changes.

> One thing I recommend to everyone, no matter their age, is that they sit down with their personal physician and plan a broader approach to managing their health than the traditional yearly physical.

The typical physical includes some good tests, such as the lipid profile. I hope you're having that done. The lipid profile looks at your total cholesterol, the HDL ("good") cholesterol and the LDL ("bad") cholesterol, the triglycerides (the blood fats), and other factors. But did you know that more than 50 percent of people who have heart attacks also had a perfectly normal lipid profile?[3] Their cholesterol was fine; their triglycerides were fine; their HDL was good; their LDL was good. So they walked away from that annual physical, saying, "I'm good. I don't need to worry; my cholesterol is great. The doctor just gave me an A! I don't need to make all those lifestyle changes."

And, of course, in today's mindset, the risk for heart disease is almost totally about cholesterol, right? Actually, as we will see, that's not true. There are many factors far more important for our heart health than cholesterol. I would rather have high cholesterol my whole life and be on a good diet and exercise program, than to have low cholesterol and eat poorly and not exercise. I guarantee you that those who follow good health practices will be healthier than those who don't—even if they struggle with some of the traditional risk factors.

Too many people resign themselves to health problems by saying, "That's just the way it is. My family history, my genetic makeup, has predetermined me to have this or that problem." That is simply not true. Medical research today in the area of genetics and epigenetics is telling us that we all have hope. We all have the potential to actually conquer the challenge of our genes.

DAVID'S STORY

I want to tell you the story of a patient of mine, a patient I'll call "David" (we met him at the beginning of this chapter). David was the resident manager of a large island resort; some people would say he had it all. He lived in a penthouse suite overlooking a beautiful turquoise bay. David was also responsible for more than 400 employees, but something was amiss. He just didn't feel right. His family doctor found that he had extremely high blood pressure; he wasn't handling stress very well. So his doctor started him on blood pressure medications.

In spite of these medications, David was still having problems. His blood pressure wasn't responding, and he was still under a lot of stress. One day he got into a dispute with one of his middle managers. Now, David is a big, strong guy—6'5," 330 pounds, a former football player. As he related the incident to me later, he said, "I became so frustrated with this guy that I was actually getting ready to slug him." When he felt himself starting to shake all over, he managed to step back from the situation. It occurred to him that he might lose his job if he didn't control his temper. With all that was going on in his life medically, this incident caused David to realize that things had to change and that he needed some additional help.

The morning after this confrontation happened, I was in my office. There had been a cancellation earlier, and I was thinking, "Good! I'll have a chance to clear my desk and catch up on all the things I have to do before the weekend."

Just then, my nurse put her head in the door and said, "Dr. Youngberg, your patient is here."

"What patient?" I asked.

David walked into my office and introduced himself. "This morning," he began, "not more than an hour or so ago, I called your clinic. I had no idea I would be able to get an appointment so fast!" There was a divine element to this; God knew David needed to be seen right away and had worked it out. He began to tell me about what had happened the day before.

"Doc," he continued, "Last night I was up in my penthouse suite with my wife and little daughter. I was sitting at my desk with my head in my hands. I didn't realize it, but my whole body was shaking. I was thinking about what had happened earlier in the day—how I was just a split second away from losing my job and destroying my reputation and my career. As I was considering what in the world I was going to do about all this, I felt a little hand come up around my shoulder, and I heard a whisper in my ear, 'Daddy, I don't want you to die!' "

David, this big former football player, was telling me this with tears starting to roll down his face.

He said, "That broke my heart. My beautiful 5-year-old daughter thought I was going to die. And you know, I could have. If I don't figure out what's going on, I'm not going to be around much longer. I'm going to have a stroke. I'm going to do something foolish, and then my family is going to be embarrassed."

Fortunately, I was starting a comprehensive lifestyle and wellness program that very weekend. It's amazing how some things work out. God had a plan.

I said, "David, we can work this out. Let's get all your labs done. And you need to come to the lifestyle program that I'm beginning this weekend."

We did a full lab work up on him—lipids, a four-hour glucose tolerance test, everything. He weighed 332 pounds; his blood pressure was 140/100 with medication. A total cholesterol of 246 put him in "heart attack alley." At 183, his unhealthy LDL cholesterol was super high; ideally, it should have been under 100. The healthy cholesterol, the HDL, was 34, and anything under 45 for men represents an independent risk for cardiovascular disease. His triglycerides—the blood fats—were 144. A triglyceride level of less than 150 is the initial goal, but less than 100 is optimal. It should have been less than 100. His fasting blood sugar levels were only four points away from full-blown diabetes. His fasting insulin, which ideally should have been less than 7, was 17, making him very insulin resistant. Insulin resistance is actually one of the most important factors driving one's personal risk not only for diabetes, but also for heart disease, cancer, headaches, infertility, and autoimmune disease. David's cardiac CRP (C-reactive protein), one of the best measures of systemic body-wide inflammation, was very high at 7. The CRP is a far more important indicator of heart attack risk than high cholesterol.

In short, David's lab tests showed he was a medical mess.

"David," I said as we reviewed his test results, "why don't we write down some goals?"

He replied, "I'm way ahead of you," and handed me a sheet of paper listing three succinct goals. The first was to weigh less than 200 pounds. To reach that goal he would have to lose more than 130 pounds! My initial impulse was to say, "That's a real long-term goal. Maybe you should start with something more short-term." But these were his goals, so I just said, "Okay, what is your next goal?"

"I want to run a marathon!"

He had just finished telling me that his knees hurt all the time. I didn't think running a marathon was a good idea or a realistic goal. But I replied, "Okay. We'll come up with a plan to help you do that."

His third goal was to become the general manager of a five-star resort in Hawaii.

Sunday afternoon David was at the opening meeting of my lifestyle wellness program. He paid attention; he took notes. He attended every meeting. You see, David understood something that many people never figure out. He understood that you must be the one in charge of your personal health. I can't do it for you. Your personal physician can't do it for you. No one can do it, except you. And if you don't do it, you won't become healthy. It's as simple as that. It's all about what you do, the choices you make. You control your genetic potential.

David radically changed his diet. He did not take baby steps. In my opinion, the research is clear. Making small changes to your diet here and there, results in minor changes in your health that are hardly noticeable. It you want to do it right, just do it!

In addition to overhauling his diet, David began a walking-jogging program. About a week later, I met him walking past my office. "Hey, Doc!" he called out. "Forget about those anti-anxiety meds. I feel great!"

What a transformation! Let me suggest to you that if you are willing to understand what works, to get involved and do what it takes, you, too, can start feeling great. Or at least, you can start feeling much better within days. Your actual risk of a stroke or a heart attack is not determined by what happened last year or two years ago or five years ago. It's largely determined by what's going on in your lifestyle and your daily environment over the last two or three days. That's good news! That means if you make a change now, your risk factors immediately plummet. If you start eating a first-class diet—the kinds of foods that generate first-class health—you will experience much better health. And I don't mean only that you will be able to look at a blood test, for example, and say, "The numbers are better, so I guess I'm healthier." No! You'll feel better. Physically and emotionally, you'll feel better.

By the second week of the program, David had lost eleven pounds. He was able to work with his personal physician to completely discontinue his blood pressure medications. His cholesterol dropped 54 points. In two weeks! It doesn't take three months to lower your cholesterol. It takes two or three weeks. David's overall blood lipids, his triglycerides, dropped by 50 percent.

But David still wasn't satisfied, because he realized that a wellness program isn't a matter of; "It's been two weeks and I'm doing better, so I can go back to living my usual life." It's a matter of changing your lifestyle for the better—for good!

David started exercising twice a day. I didn't tell him to do that, but he decided, "If I'm going to run a marathon, I'd better start putting in some miles. So he gradually worked up to walking and jogging forty-five minutes twice a day. He was on call 24/7 as the resident manager of a 1,200-room resort. If he could find the time to exercise forty-five minutes twice a day, I suspect anyone can. By the way, I'm not suggesting you need to exercise forty-five minutes twice a day. But you do need to figure out how exercise fits into your health goals and come up with a plan that's reasonable for you.

David not only began eating better, he learned portion control. After all, he had 130 pounds or so to lose to reach his goal. Portion control was vital. Within six months, he lost 79 pounds and lowered his cholesterol even further. He was no longer prediabetic. His fasting insulin was back to normal, and his cardiac CRP, the measure of inflammation, had dropped by 50 percent. David still hadn't met any of his three goals. But look at how much he'd accomplished. Look at the positive progression. And this highlights another important point: Don't become discouraged about not reaching your goals as long as you're experiencing steady improvement.

A year and a half went by. During this time, I would see David from time to time for consultations. Then one day I was in an airport, returning home from California, when I saw David and his wife and daughter walking toward me on the concourse. It was obvious that he'd reached his first goal. He looked lean and mean, healthy and fit!

"David!" I said, "What are you doing here?"

"I lost all that weight," he replied. "And guess what I did a week ago?"

"You didn't!" I answered.

"Yes, I did. I ran the Honolulu marathon. I did it in four hours and thirty minutes!" Not a world record, but it was a major accomplishment for David. "And you haven't heard the best news of all," he continued. "We're moving to Maui." I remembered David's third goal—to become the general manager of a world-class resort.

YOUR CHOICES MATTER

What motivates you? What is it that makes you want to change? Why are you reading this book? I want you to write it out in words and save it for future reference. Write down exactly how you feel right now. Write out all your family history. Write out your goals and some ideas for achieving them. If you need help doing this, you can go to my clinic's website, dryoungberg.com, and it will show you how to write out your family history, your personal history, all your health concerns.

Why do I want you to do this? Because I frequently work with people who tell me after two or three months, "I don't really feel any different. This isn't working." But I have all the records in my computer, all the things they wrote down at the beginning. And I start reading it back to them—how they used to feel. You see, when we get into the new "normal" and we feel so much better, we begin to forget how things used to be. We begin to think that this is how we've always felt. So document where you are now—not just your lab results, but also what is going on subjectively in your life. What are you eating? What are you doing for exercise? How are you feeling physically, emotionally, spiritually? Document these things. Set reasonable goals and pay attention to them.

> You have roughly 20,000 genes that control everything in your body. But it's the frontal lobe in your brain that controls those 20,000 genes. The choices you make and the thoughts you have affect those genes directly and indirectly. You have that power.

AN OPERATOR'S MANUAL FOR HEALTHFUL LIVING

Chronic disease and health dysfunction is most often caused by a deficiency of some kind. There are two aspects to health: (1) avoiding those things that tear down the body, and (2) making sure we're taking in enough of those things that build up the body. If you don't have enough of the right nutrients, even miniscule amounts of toxins will affect your health negatively. We need to have enough of the right things. So the first step to health and wellness is eating a first-class diet. That's the topic of the next chapter. Hippocrates said it best thousands of years ago: "Let foods be your medicine and medicine be your food."[4] Hippocrates is considered to be the father of modern medicine. But there's another Father who is far more important than Hippocrates, and that is our heavenly Father, our Creator.

This Creator has given us an operator's manual for living—the Bible. In the very beginning, God said, "See, I have given you every herb that yields seed . . . and every tree whose fruit yields seed; to you it shall be for food." Our Creator gave us an understanding of what is best for optimizing our epigenome, and we're just now starting to understand how that works. Risk is determined by the epigenetic changes that reflect our *exposome*—all the things that actually activate our genes for good or bad. Our exposome is all the things in our environment. It's all the choices we make. It's all the lifestyle behaviors in which we participate. It's what we eat, what we drink, what we think, and what we do. That is our exposome.

So you want to choose colorful, natural foods that change the exposome. Lots of good colorful foods. That's the first step. You want to make sure that at least 80 percent of your diet comes from whole plant-based foods. The average American is getting less than 10 percent, and that includes french fries as vegetables! Don't follow the Standard American Diet (SAD diet). That diet is guaranteed to create an exposome that will destroy your genetic potential.

WHO'S IN CHARGE?

Who is in charge? Who makes the decisions that affect your genes? Remember, it all starts in the brain—in the choices you make. That's why we will be focusing throughout this book on attitudes, emotions, and values. It's these things that influence choices, and choices influence everything else. You can modify your genes. There are studies showing that lifestyle choices can dramatically turn on and turn off genes in the right direction in just three months. I believe that our genetic expression can change very, very quickly. It reminds me of the statement by the apostle Paul. "Do not be conformed to this world, but be transformed by the renewing of your mind."[5] In other words, don't follow what other people are doing just because it's the norm. The norm today in our modern, fast-paced, stress-filled society is not conducive to health. Today, it's considered "normal" to have heart disease, diabetes, or even cancer. I'm not saying that bad things don't happen to people who live a healthful lifestyle. They do. But you have the opportunity to dramatically improve your health by paying attention to Paul's counsel. It's not just spiritual advice; it reflects physiological reality. You can experience transformational change in your health and wellness by making positive choices every day that will lead you to your ultimate goal of good health.

Don't sit on the sidelines and let your doctor or nurse or others member of your healthcare team make all the decisions. That's not their job. Their job is to give you information and awareness and then let you choose. You need to make changes in your life if you're going to become healthier. Your doctor can't do that for you. If your genes are the cards that you're dealt, then epigenetics is how you play them. Seneca, a Roman orator around the time of Christ, said, "It is part of the cure to wish to be cured."

In the chapters ahead you'll learn about a number of specific lifestyle choices you can make and how to put them into practice in your life. But an important part of the cure is that you have to really want it. And not just for one day or one week or a few months. You've got to want it for life.

You can choose a new direction. Everything depends on the right action of the will. Everything depends upon the choices that you make. Through the right exercise of the will, dramatic changes can take place in your life and in your health! Are you ready?

In the next chapter, we'll be looking at exercise and diet, two of the most important areas where changes can really pay off in improving your levels of health and wellness.

CHAPTER SUMMARY

>> The environment in which you live, the choices you make, and the habits you form all greatly affect how your genes function.

>> The function of our genes and their expression can be changed. You can actually turn off many of your bad genes and turn on your good genes.

>> Family history is not the most important factor in determining your risk of disease. In fact, it is one of the least important.

>> Transformational change can take place in your health by implementing appropriate lifestyle and nutritional strategies.

>> Your exposome is all the things in your environment that influence genetic expression. It's the choices you make, your lifestyle, what you eat, drink, think, and do.

>> It is never too late to begin making changes that will transform your health.

>> At least 80 percent of your diet should come from whole plant-based foods.

>> Your choices matter. Everything depends on the right action of the will.

ENDNOTES

1   Jirtle, R, "Transposable Elements: Targets for Early Nutritional Effects on Epigenetic Gene Regulation," Molecular and Cellular Biology, 23 (2003) 5293–5300.

2   Eddy, D, "Relationship of Insulin Resistance and Related Metabolic Variables to Coronary Artery Disease: A Mathematical Analysis," Diabetes Care, 32 (2009), 361-366.

3   Ridker, P., et al., "Rosuvastatin to Prevent Vascular Events in Men and Women With Elevated C-Reactive Protein," New England Journal of Medicine, 2008; 359: 2195-2207.

4   Genesis 1:29, NKJV.

5   Romans 12:2, NKJV.

— TWO —

Calories In, Calories Out

THE IMPORTANCE OF DIET AND EXERCISE

IF YOU'RE SERIOUS ABOUT REACHING YOUR FULL genetic potential for health and wellness, you've got to be serious about exercise and diet. These are two critical components of an effective wellness program. The choices we make concerning exercise and diet have been extensively researched in terms of how they affect the way our genes function. As we saw in the previous chapter, the genes you were born with are not unchangeable; they are not fixed indicators of how healthy you can be. The genes themselves do not determine risk. It's whether or not a certain gene is turned on or turned off. Risk is determined by these epigenetic changes that reflect our *exposome*.

And what is our exposome? As we saw in the previous chapter, it's all the things in our environment. It's all the choices we make. It's all the lifestyle behaviors we participate in. It's what we eat, what we drink, what we think, and what we do. That is our exposome. These are the things that actually activate our genes for good or for bad. By turning off "bad" genes and turning on "good" genes you have the potential to literally master your own genetic health. Exercise and diet are two of the primary ways you can affect positive change in the expression of your genes.

Unfortunately, a large segment of society today is following a diet made up mostly of highly processed food, food that can be prepared quickly. We call this fast food and junk food. A poor diet is influencing their genetic destiny—not because they have bad genes, but because their diet is turning on the "bad" genes. We need to understand far better than we do that our future risk of disease depends to a great degree on the food that is sitting on our plate.

Also, unfortunately, a large portion of society today gets little meaningful or effective exercise. In this chapter, we're going to be looking at how diet and exercise are related and the importance of a balanced relationship between them for increasing our health and wellness levels.

In the United States and in many other countries around the world, there has been an obvious and increasing problem with overweight and obesity. This problem affects all age groups. It is a clear example of what happens when there is an imbalance between diet and exercise.

BALANCING EXERCISE AND DIET FOR WEIGHT LOSS

For many people, the number one health-related goal is to lose weight. Now, setting goals is important. But they need to be specific, measurable goals. "I want to lose weight" isn't really a goal. It's too general, too undefined. "I want to lose thirty pounds, from 196 to 166, over the next six months," is a goal. Maybe weight is not an issue with you at all. Maybe your goal is: "I want to improve my blood pressure from 140/90 to 120/80 so that when I meet with my family doctor in three months I may be able to stop taking certain medications." Those are specific, measurable goals.

> Of course, it's not enough just to set a goal. You need to develop a plan for how you can actually achieve that goal. You have to figure out the most effective way to get there.

Let's say your goal is to lose two pounds in a week. What would it take to do that? What is the most effective way to reach that goal? Both exercise and diet can cause weight loss. Which should you focus on in order to lose weight most effectively?

I faced that question nearly thirty years ago during my final doctoral defense before my committee chairman, department professors, and visiting professors.

Things seemed to be coming to a close, and I actually thought the formal session was over. Then, seemingly out of the blue, one of the visiting professors asked, "What's the most effective way to lose weight—exercise or diet?"

The question took me by surprise a bit. And since I've always been an exercise guy, I replied without thinking, "Exercise. I believe exercise is the most important strategy for weight loss."

My committee chairman looked at me when I said that, and the look on his face told me he didn't agree. But instead of making me look bad and embarrassing me, he said, "Why don't we go through the mathematics of what it takes to lose two pounds in a week, using exercise versus doing the same with diet?"

So we did. You might be interested in the numbers and the final conclusion.

First, how many calories are there in a pound of fat? The answer is 3,500 calories. That means that the energy in a pound of fat is pretty concentrated. It's almost as if the human body wasn't designed to burn up that much fat very quickly. Why? Because we were initially designed not to have a lot of fat. So we're programmed to conserve the fat we have.

If there are 3,500 calories in a pound of fat, how many are there in two pounds? This isn't too difficult; it's about third-grade math. Obviously, there are 7,000 calories in two pounds of fat. And if you want to lose those 7,000 calories in one week, you would need to lose 1,000 calories each day. Walking, running, jogging, etc. burns up an average of 100 calories per mile. So to lose 7,000 calories (two pounds) of fat in a week using exercise, you would need to walk, run, or jog seventy miles—ten miles a day, every day for a week.

Now don't misunderstand. I'm not trying to discourage you from using exercise as part of your wellness program. I'm trying to help you understand that there is a physiological difference, a major difference, between using exercise solely as a form of weight loss versus using diet as the main source of weight loss.

Let's take a look at how effective diet might be as a means of losing that same two pounds in a week. How many snacks or unnecessary food portions would you need to eliminate on a regular, daily basis in order to accomplish the very same thing?

Most typical snacks contain about 250 calories. Many, obviously, have many more calories than that. But using 250 calories as an average, we would need to eliminate four snacks a day in order to lose 1,000 calories. Using exercise, those same 1,000 calories required ten miles of walking, running, or jogging.

> What's the take-home message? The message is that diet is much more effective in addressing weight control than is exercise.

It is much easier and less time consuming to avoid eating four snacks than it is to walk or run ten miles. If you have to choose just one method, it's clearly easier to lose weight by avoiding unnecessary food items than it is to lose weight by exercising.

BALANCING EXERCISE AND DIET FOR FITNESS AND OVERALL HEALTH

When I was in college, my dad decided one day that I should paint the hallway of our house. So while I was painting, I was listening to the radio—WBBM, Chicago News Radio. Back in the early 80s, Bob and Betty Sanders were co-hosts of a talk show on that station. So I was painting and listening, when the announcer said, "At the top of the hour, Bob and Betty Sanders will be talking to Jim Fixx, an avid runner and marathoner who is promoting a race here in Chicago."

As soon as I heard the name, Jim Fixx, I started paying closer attention. The year before, my father had given me Fixx's book on running; it had a picture of his legs on the cover—muscular, lean, fit. The book was all about how to stay motivated and involved in an exercise program. I was into exercise, so I was very interested in hearing this interview with Jim Fixx.

The first question Betty Sanders asked was this: "Jim, I understand you run ten miles every day." She paused for effect and then asked, "What kind of crazy, radical person would take the time to run ten miles every day? Why do you do that?"

Without missing a beat, Jim said, "Well, when I run ten miles a day, I can eat anything I want."

It was an awesome comeback. But even then, I immediately realized that there was a big problem with what Jim had just said. The problem is that you can't just eat anything you want. Not if you want to be healthy. It's not a question of weight. Although almost everybody is interested in their weight and focused on their weight, the main issue affecting wellness negatively is not weight. It really never has been.

> Of course, there is nothing wrong with setting goals for appropriate weight loss—or weight gain as the case may be. But just because a person is lean, without an ounce of excess fat on their body, in no way suggests that that person is fully healthy.

So when Jim Fixx made that comment about being able to eat anything he wanted as long as he exercised, I remember saying out loud, "Jim, you're going to have problems." I wasn't a lifestyle medicine specialist or a nutritionist at that time, but I intuitively understood Jim's comment didn't add up.

Two years later I was in my first year of professional training at Loma Linda University in southern California. One day, I was headed home in my car after my last class, when I heard on the news that Jim Fixx, long-distance runner and author of many books on running, had been found dead that morning. Halfway through his daily ten-mile run he had collapsed and died. The running world, the fitness world, was stunned. How could Jim Fixx, someone who seemed so fit, die of a massive heart attack?

The first thing that crossed my mind when I heard of his death was that comment he had made two years earlier on the radio: "When I run ten miles a day, I can eat anything I want." In one sense, that statement was true. When he exercised that much, Jim didn't have to worry about what he ate in terms of weight. He was burning off any extra weight he was gaining from what he ate. No problem. But when it comes to cardiovascular risk, it doesn't work that way. You can't just burn off cardiovascular risk. You can burn off some of it, but you can't burn off most of it.

Cholesterol, after all, is not a caloric substance. It's a waxy substance that, in excess and associated with other toxic molecules, can infiltrate the artery wall, stimulating an inflammatory reaction that leads to significant atheroma or plaque buildup. That's the cause of heart disease. That's the cause of stroke risk.

REPLACING BAD HABITS WITH GOOD HABITS

Jim Fixx's story also illustrates the way good habits can push out bad ones.

When Jim was in his early 20s, his father died of a massive heart attack. Jim became depressed. He went from being a high school and college athlete to being a couch potato. He began drinking multiple beers every night and smoking several packs of cigarettes a day.

One day a friend from his younger days said, "Jim, there is a 10K run coming up. Why don't we train for it and do it together?" So Jim agreed. As he was training for this 10K run, he noticed that he began feeling better. The depression was starting to lift. He had more energy. As he became more involved in running, he asked himself, "Why am I smoking? I'm not going to be able to run my best if I'm smoking." So he gave up smoking.

And he didn't give up smoking just because it was bad for his running. He quit smoking because he didn't feel the need to smoke in the same way he had before. You see, when you are doing something good for yourself physically, it helps manage stress in your life. And if smoking, for example, is your strategy for managing stress, now you don't have the need to smoke.

There's an important health principle involved here. It's very difficult to give up something bad for you, unless you first replace it with something good that is equally effective at providing whatever satisfaction you were getting from the bad habit. That's what makes exercise such an extremely powerful tool to help people give up their addictions.

CALORIES IN, CALORIES OUT

Jim Fixx became a good friend of Dr. Kenneth Cooper of the Aerobics Institute in Dallas, Texas. Dr. Cooper was famous for his work with the Dallas

Cowboys. Coach Tom Landry was upset that his Cowboys were falling apart during the fourth quarter. He called in Dr. Cooper and asked, "What do we need to do?"

After analyzing the situation, Dr. Cooper told the coach, "All these guys are doing is getting buff with weights. They're never going to last more than two or three quarters. They need to start exercising longer distances in an aerobic exercise program." After Cooper began working with the team, the Dallas Cowboys became known as "The Fourth Quarter Team," the team that would always come back late in the game and win.

I had the privilege in 1976 of listening to Dr. Cooper give a lecture about exercise at Andrews University in southwestern Michigan. At the end of the presentation, someone asked him, "Dr. Cooper, what about diet? Does it matter what you eat?"

Authoritatively, Dr. Cooper replied, "As long as your exercise output in calories equals your caloric input in food calories, you're good."

But when Jim Fixx died, Dr. Cooper began thinking about the idea that it doesn't really matter what you eat as long as you balance it with sufficient exercise to prevent weight gain. You see, that idea has never actually been true; he just didn't know it at the time.

Dr. Cooper started paying attention to nutrition. He wrote the book, *Running Without Fear,* because after Jim Fixx's death, many had become afraid to run. They said, "You've got to have a doctor's appointment before you start an exercise program."

Dr. Cooper said that it is ridiculous to think that anytime you do something healthy you should first get clearance from your doctor! We need to be exercising more and exercising more often, he said, but not necessarily exercising strenuously for lengthy periods of time.

BALANCING EXERCISE AND DIET FOR HEALTH RISKS

About this time, Dr. Cooper hired Dr. Roy Vartabedian, a colleague and a friend of mine, to run his Lifestyle Medicine Center. Dr. Vartabedian introduced the important concept of controlling cardiovascular risks, and health risks in general, with a balanced approach of nutrition and exercise. His book, *Nutripoints,* was a best seller that showed you how to choose the foods that will have the greatest impact on your ability to change your genes in positive directions.

Jim Fixx probably extended his life many years by exercising on a regular basis. Sadly, however, he might still be around today, even continuing to run ten miles a day, if he had known what we know now about the power of diet and the importance of balancing exercise and nutrition.

I'm frequently asked which is more important—exercise or diet—in terms of overall health risks and wellness. My answer is, "The most important is the one you're not doing. That's the most important one." You need to have both good nutrition and a good exercise program in your life. Both are important wellness strategies that are critical to your health.

We know that simply by exercising on a regular basis you can cut your risk of having a heart attack by 50 percent.[1, 2] And if you do have a heart attack, regular exercise increases your potential to fully recover from that heart attack by another 70 percent. It does this by stimulating collateral circulation—the growth and development of new blood vessels to feed areas that may not be receiving an adequate blood supply.[3] So exercise is a powerful wellness strategy.

Exercise also lowers blood fats. It naturally increases the good (HDL) cholesterol, the kind that sucks the plaque out of the arteries and moves it to the liver where the liver can get rid of it. By the way, the best thing you can do to help the liver get rid of toxic LDL cholesterol is to make sure that every meal you eat has at least ten, and preferably fifteen, grams of whole-food fiber. Doing this will force you to eat a lot of whole, plant-based foods, because animal products of any kind contain zero fiber. You will have to focus on what I call "first-class" foods.

Another benefit of exercise is that it dramatically improves digestion.[4, 5] We'll be looking at digestion in detail in Chapter 5. Digestion is critical to good health. Without good digestion, you're simply not going to be healthy, and your body will age faster. Your body must efficiently absorb the nutrients, vitamins, minerals, and other phyto-nutrients in your food if you expect to be healthy.

Light, moderate exercise immediately after a meal can dramatically improve digestion[6] and potentially enhance absorption of key micro-nutrients. I'm not talking about exercise that will make you huff and puff. But a short walk after eating is one of the most powerful strategies for improving digestion.

> Exercise is also extremely beneficial for anyone who struggles with out-of-control blood sugar. A diabetic or prediabetic individual can lower his or her blood sugar anywhere from one to three points for every minute spent walking immediately after finishing a meal.

Why immediately? Because if you wait an hour after eating to walk, your blood sugar will have already reached its peak; it is already starting to damage the body. So walk immediately after eating. This will not only dramatically blunt your peak in blood sugar, it will also decrease the risk of your blood sugar dropping too rapidly two, three, or four hours later. Light exercise after eating helps balance your blood sugar nicely.

This is important because of the prevalence of diabetes today. By age 40 to 59, one out of two already has prediabetes. Most of those who are prediabetic don't realize it; that's why testing is so important. The test needs to be a glucose tolerance test—a fasting blood sugar test is often inadequate. For those between the ages of 60 and 74, two out of three are at least prediabetic. Over age 75, it's three out of four—a 75 percent chance of being at least prediabetic.[7] The insulin resistance syndrome associated with prediabetes and diabetes is the number one risk factor for premature heart disease.[8] Exercise at any time of the day is beneficial in controlling blood sugar levels.

Statin medications are often prescribed to lower inflammation and thus help prevent plaque buildup within the artery walls. But did you know that exercise has been shown to be as effective in lowering inflammation as a statin medicine?[9] Either an optimal diet or exercise program can independently lower inflammation as well as—and often better than—cholesterol-lowering medications.[10, 11] But in my years of clinical experience, combining all the wellness strategies will, on average, lower the cardiac CRP inflammation by 50 percent in just two to three weeks time.

EXERCISE AND FEELINGS OF WELLNESS

When something's wrong in our lives, when something is missing and we're not at ease, what often happens? Often our eating habits take a turn for the worse. Subconsciously, we begin asking ourselves, "What can I eat that will change the way I feel? I want to feel better." And when we start feeling that way, chances are we're going to make food choices that aren't very good for us. I know; I've been there.

Exercise has a powerful ability to change the way you feel. Exercise is such a crucial part of wellness program, that I'm convinced that if you aren't exercising, you're probably not eating effectively either. Why? Because exercise is what gives you that feeling of wellness that allows you to eat those foods that optimize genetic expression even further.

PLANNING AND CHOICES—A PERSONAL STORY

Let me tell you a little story about myself. Between 1994 and 2008 I was living in Guam, serving as the Director of the Lifestyle Medicine Clinic. Almost every evening, I was conducting a program of some kind. One was a six-month program called NEWSTART that focused on intensive lifestyle medicine strategies. We did comprehensive lab work on those participating in the program—at the beginning, at two weeks, and then at three months and six months. We knew exactly what was going on with the participants' lab work. We checked blood sugar every day before and after meals, and before and after exercise. We figured out optimal meal plans and exercise programs for each individual. I mention all this to let you know that I was very much aware of effective strategies for health and wellness.

I love to play basketball and normally played at lunchtime on Tuesdays and Thursdays. But one particular week, I got caught up in meetings at the clinic and missed my basketball days. Then I got busy in other work and ended up going a whole week without any significant exercise. Oh, I got a little exercise going for walks with my patients, but not the type of exercise that I really needed.

After a week of very little activity and no real exercise, I got up early on Sunday morning and went to play basketball. I was looking forward to playing. I was stir crazy. I needed some exercise. I enjoyed it so much that instead of playing for just an hour as I usually did, I played for three hours.

Full court basketball, hardcore basketball! By the time I finished playing, I was famished, drenched in sweat, and exhausted.

I went home, ate a meal, and rehydrated myself. Twenty minutes later, I was back at the refrigerator. I didn't feel satisfied. Something was missing. The first thing I knew, I was eating more food, even though I had just eaten twenty minutes earlier. I barely had time to begin digesting the food I had eaten only a few minutes before. But I was insatiable.

The rest of the day I was essentially worthless. My wife was upset with me, because I wasn't crossing off any of the little jobs on her honey-do list. I just lay on the couch and watched football and slept, because I was so exhausted. But every forty-five minutes or so, I would get up and find myself back at the refrigerator. I didn't really care what I ate at that point; I just wanted to eat something.

The next night, Monday night, I had a lifestyle medicine lecture to give. The clinic chef had prepared a wonderful meal for the whole group of patients. I got my meal and ate it. I enjoyed it, but after finishing, I was still feeling unsatisfied.

Tuesday night came around. For three days I had been eating and eating and eating. It seemed I couldn't feel satisfied. That night I was to give a presentation on nutrition and the importance of eating first-class foods. My chef, knowing that patients would want to talk to me afterward and that I probably wouldn't be able to eat for a while after the presentation, prepared a meal for me ahead of time. "Dr. Youngberg," she said, "here's your meal. Go ahead and eat it now before your lecture."

So I ate the meal she had prepared. Then I gave my presentation. The patients listened, took notes, and seemed to appreciate the information. Following the program, they went through line for the meal that had been prepared for them. I was able to talk with many of them and discuss issues further. About an hour and a half later, the chef came up to me and said, "I can tell you're still hungry by the way you're looking at the food in the back. Here's another plate."

I ate another plate of food! Shortly after eating that second dinner, I was driving home. By this time it was probably 8:30 or 9:00 o'clock. Marine Corps Drive is a major highway on Guam. There are three lanes in each direction, with a center turn lane—seven lanes in all. I always drove in the far right lane so I could look to the right and see the beautiful bay shimmering in the moonlight. That night I was looking at the moonlight, when all at once, out of the corner of my eye, I caught the reflection of another light—to the left.

That other light was a Dairy Queen® sign! I had never noticed it before, but instantly my mind flashed back thirty years. I saw myself as a 12-year-old, riding my bike to the local Dairy Queen to get a Peanut Buster® Parfait.

> I turned the car across seven lanes of traffic, bounced into the driveway, parked, and walked in. "Do you still make Peanut Buster Parfaits?" I asked the young girl behind the counter. "We certainly do," she answered.

I was salivating while she made it! I hadn't had one in years; I hadn't even thought of one in years. But when it arrived, I slurped it down in less than two minutes, enjoying every gooey, sweet bite. Within another minute or two, I was starting to feel a head rush, and I began asking myself, What just happened? I'm a wellness doctor. I just finished giving a lecture on nutrition to people who look to me as someone who knows what he is talking about! I outlined a nutritional plan for them to follow. What in the world happened?

I could beat myself up about the poor willpower that I showed that night. But it really wasn't a question of willpower; it was a question of poor planning. This is a very important principle. I had failed to plan and follow a proper exercise program throughout the week. Then I had done something even more stupid by exercising vigorously, exhaustively for several hours in a row. Should I have expected that my body was going to just bounce back and be okay with all that I had done to it?

If you or I don't plan a proper exercise program—and then follow that plan—we shouldn't be surprised if our bodies rebel. When we put the body through trauma, we tend to lose control.

FOLLOWING THE PLAN CONSISTENTLY

You see, the frontal lobe was placed in our brain so that we would be able to exercise control. It's critical that we make good choices and put ourselves in position to exercise self control when faced with temptations. Consistently following your wellness program is extremely critical. It's not enough to approach wellness as an "on-again, off-again" affair. In fact, you may be shortening your life by doing that. You may be increasing your risk for a heart attack or stroke. Wellness depends on developing a plan and consistently following it day in and day out.

Sometimes you have to say no to things you really, really want to do, in order to say yes to things you know are much more important. Setting limits is not hugely popular in today's society, but I would suggest to you that if you really want to enjoy optimal health, you have to become good at setting limits for yourself. In any walk of life, those who are the most successful, the most effective, are those who understand how to set limits for themselves. For more information about how to set limits on your diet and develop a tasty First Class Diet Plan, see the Appendix. If you can learn to follow your wellness plan consistently, I guarantee that you will be able to reach your goals over time.

CHAPTER SUMMARY

>>   Exercise done properly can powerfully change how you feel, improve your mood, and significantly decrease your cravings for snacks and excess calories.

>>   There is an obvious and increasing international problem with obesity associated with poor diet and lack of exercise.

>>   When considering calories eaten versus calories burned off—diet is much more effective in addressing weight loss than is exercise.

>>   Good habits can push out bad habits.

>>   Regular exercise can reduce your risk of having a heart attack by 50 percent.

>>   Wellness depends on developing a plan and following it consistently day in and day out.

>>   Sometimes you have to say no to things you really want to do in order to say yes to things you know are much more important.

ENDNOTES

1   Ades, P., "Cardiac Rehabilitation and Secondary Prevention of Coronary Heart Disease," *New England Journal of Medicine*, 2001; 345:892-902.

2   Manson, J., "Walking Compared with Vigorous Exercise for the Prevention of Cardiovascular Events in Women," *New England Journal of Medicine*, 2002; 347:716-725.

3   Uhlemann, M., "Impact of Different Exercise Training Modalities on the Coronary Collateral Circulation and Plaque Composition in Patients with Significant Coronary Artery Disease (EXCITE Trial): Study Protocol for a Randomized Controlled Trial," *Trials*, 2012, 13:167.

4   Rissanen, A.; Fogelholm, M., "Physical Activity in the Prevention and Treatment of Other Morbid Conditions and Impairments Associated with Obesity: Current Evidence and Research Issues." *Medicine & Science in Sports & Exercise*, 31:S635–S645.

5   Leitzmann, M. F.; Rimm, E. B.; Willett, W. C.; et al., "Recreational Physical Activity and the Risk of Cholecystectomy in Women," *New England Journal of Medicine*, 341:777–784.

6   Franke, A., "Postprandial Walking but not Consumption of Alcoholic Digestifs or Espresso Accelerates Gastric Emptying in Healthy Volunteers," *Journal of Gastrointestinal Liver Disease*, March 2008, vol. 17, no. 1, 27-31.

7   Cowie, C., et al., "Full Accounting of Diabetes and Pre-Diabetes in the U.S. Population in 1988-1994 and 2005-2006," *Diabetes Care*, 32 (2009) 287–294.

8   *Diabetes Care*, vol. 32, no. 2, February, 2009.

9   Geffken, D., et al., "Association Between Physical Activity and Markers of Inflammation in a Healthy Elderly Population," *American Journal of Epidemiology*, 2001; 153:242-250.

10 Jenkins, D. J., et al. "Effects of a Dietary Portfolio of Cholesterol-Lowering Foods vs Lovastatin on Serum Lipids and C-Reactive Protein." JAMA, July 23/30, 2003; 290:502–510.

11 Church, T. S., et al., "Associations Between Cardiorespiratory Fitness and C-Reactive Protein in Men," *Arteriosclerosis, Thrombosis, and Vascular Biology*, November 1, 2002; 22:1869-1876.

—THREE—

Matters
of the Heart
OPTIMIZING CIRCULATION
AND HEART HEALTH

DOES "OPTIMIZING CIRCULATION" SOUND BORING? It might. Until you realize that circulation involves every organ system in the body. Until you realize that you can't really be healthy without good circulation. No organ system will be healthy if it doesn't have an adequate blood supply circulating to that area. So it's extremely important that we take care of our circulatory system.

In your automobile you have a water pump that circulates coolant throughout the engine to keep it from overheating. In your home, a pump provides the pressure to circulate water through the plumbing. It's the same in your body. A pump circulates blood throughout your body to all the organs and systems. The main pump doing this, of course, is your heart. But it doesn't do it all by itself.

HOW EXERCISE HELPS CIRCULATION

One of the great benefits of exercise is that it puts into motion a multitude of pumps that help the heart circulate blood more efficiently. Every single muscle in your body is able to assist the heart in pumping blood through the circulatory system and eventually back to the heart again. Without this help, the heart not only has to pump blood to all the tissues, it then has to push all that blood back up to the heart itself. That's a tremendous load on the heart. But exercise causes the muscles to act like mini-pumps, helping the heart move the blood around the body and back to the heart.

INFLAMMATION AND CIRCULATION

Clearly, we want our circulatory system to work as efficiently as possible. And inflammation is one of the big issues negatively effecting circulation.

When you hear the word *inflammation,* what comes to your mind? Most people think of a swollen, inflamed finger that has been injured somehow, or an infected sore that is red and hot. Those are certainly examples of inflammation.

But when I'm talking about inflammation having a negative effect on your circulation, I'm talking about inflammation as a systemic issue.

That's the problem with inflammation—it can be everywhere in the body in a way that isn't obvious like a swollen finger. Exercise is an excellent way to lower systemic inflammation and thus improve circulation.

A WELLNESS APPROACH TO CIRCULATION ISSUES

In this chapter, I'll be discussing circulation issues in the context of a wellness approach to evaluating and treating such things as cholesterol, insulin resistance, thyroid deficiencies, and other advanced cardiovascular or circulatory risk factors.

A short time ago, I had the opportunity to be in a small group of individuals attending a conference with Dr. Paul Ziajka, a physician and researcher who is a director of the Florida Lipid Institute. Dr. Ziajka is a lipidologist, which means that he is a specialist in helping other doctors successfully control their patients' cholesterol and lipid values. It was an invaluable opportunity for me to ask him questions for about two hours. It's very important for doctors to stay up-to-date with recent developments and findings. It's easy for a doctor to spend decades believing certain ideas and concepts, when they may have been disproven years ago—perhaps shortly after he or she learned them! So opportunities such as this with Dr. Ziajka are priceless.

FOCUSING ON HIDDEN RISK FACTORS

I want to share with you one important thing Dr. Ziajka told us at that conference:

"Sixty percent of patients who have heart attacks have completely normal lipid profiles. Their cholesterol is normal; their triglyceride blood fats are normal; their 'good' cholesterol (HDL) is normal; their 'bad' cholesterol (LDL) is normal. "

In other words, according to Dr. Ziajka, you might as well flip a coin to decide whether you're at risk for a heart attack as to rely on a traditional lipid profile."

Now don't misunderstand. I still believe a traditional lipid profile is a valuable test. It can give us a lot of information. But you have to recognize that it addresses only about 40 percent of the risk for a heart attack that an individual may have.[1] In fact, a lipid profile is not FDA approved for assessing stroke risk at all. It's designed primarily to determine risk of a heart attack. We need to go beyond the normal lipid profile to establish our heart attack risk.

One of the main problems we face as we work with assessing risk and how to deal with it is that we—both doctors and patients—become so focused on treating the risk factors identified by these traditional tests that we forget there are other areas we need to focus on as well. If the lipid profile is addressing only 40 percent of the risk of a heart attack, then there are other factors involved in the remaining 60 percent of risk. Yet we often feel that as long as we're managing cholesterol and blood fats, we're doing all we can to minimize the risk of a heart attack.

We can see this same misdirected focus in the treatment of diabetes. As I work with individuals who've had diabetes for a long time, it's becomes very clear that the management focus of their diabetes has become so all-consuming that everything is about controlling blood sugar. Of course, everyone with diabetes needs to be managing blood sugar. The accepted standards also state that their lipids need to be carefully monitored. Their blood pressure should be looked at closely and also managed. In fact, one physician who was the managing partner of a large medical group I once worked with, said in order to properly treat a person with diabetes, that person should be taking at least seven different prescription medicines, most of them related to high blood pressure, even if the person didn't have high blood pressure. They needed, he said, to be taking cholesterol lowering medications even if they didn't have high cholesterol. Why? Because the risk for cardiovascular disease, heart attacks, and strokes was so great with diabetes that the standard of care should be to aggressively manage for those risk factors.

> But the problem, again, is that those risk factors represent only a portion of the risk. So no matter how aggressively you address those risks, you're still ignoring much of the risk. And that risk could be dramatically reduced if we are aware of what that risk actually is.

So cholesterol values, triglyceride values, the ratio of "good" cholesterol to "bad" cholesterol—all these factors represent only the tip of the iceberg for risk in terms of cardiovascular disease. That "tip" is important. We need to be aware of those risk factors and try to deal effectively with them. But underneath the ocean's surface, there is this additional mammoth amount of risk that is represented by the bulk of the iceberg. I refer to this as the "metabolic mess," all the known and unknown factors, the total risk, whether you're dealing with diabetes or hypertension or cardiovascular disease or immune disorders. Whatever health concerns you have, you have to focus on that hidden risk. If you don't, you're going to miss the vast majority of the risk.

WELLNESS MEANS MORE THAN JUST BEING FIT

When I was 24 years old, I thought I was Mr. Fitness. It was about that time that doctors Brown and Goldstein won the Nobel Prize in medicine for discovering the important role that LDL cholesterol plays in causing heart disease. So I said, "I'm going to get my cholesterol checked." I was a life-long vegetarian, and I was exercising daily, so I thought my cholesterol levels would be pretty good.

Wrong! The test showed that my cholesterol levels were sky high—almost off the chart! I was above the 95th percentile. That meant that 95 percent of individuals my age had a lower cholesterol level that I did. Believe me, you don't want to have a cholesterol level that is higher than 95 percent of the people your age.

> You don't even want to have a cholesterol level that is higher than 50 percent of people your age! When it comes to cholesterol, or any other risk factor, you don't want to be "normal." Normal isn't healthy. You want to be optimally healthy, and you start toward that goal by paying attention to these risk factors.

Those off-the-chart cholesterol numbers should have been a clear message to me. You see, my grandfather died of a massive heart attack a year before I was born. He was a wonderful man, a Christian pastor. Everyone loved him. At least that's what I was told. I never had the opportunity to know my grandfather or to spend time with him. He was never, ever there for me. Why? Because he wasn't aware of his risk.

Of course, that was a long time ago. We've come a long way since then in being able to objectively and categorically figure out what our risk factors are for various diseases. We have tools and strategies that we'll be discussing throughout this book that can help us avoid suffering my grandfather's fate.

When I was in my 20s, even though I knew my grandfather had died of a heart attack, somehow I didn't really think about how that fact affected me and my heart health. Then, some years later, my uncle died of a massive heart attack. He was an ER physician in his 50s. He had just treated a patient in the ER and had returned to the little room a short distance away, where he slept. A nurse passing by found him lying face down on the floor near the open door of his room. Efforts to revive him failed. So when I discovered my cholesterol was sky high, suddenly a light came on for me, and I said to myself, *If this can happen to Uncle Gorden, maybe it could happen to me.*

A THREE-WEEK RESEARCH PROJECT

About six years after that initial cholesterol test, I was around 30 years old, practicing nutritional and lifestyle medicine at the Loma Linda University Faculty Medical Group in Sun City, California. It was a retirement community, so there were a lot of healthcare needs. Over the previous six years I had been much more careful with my diet. I had become aware that wellness is about more than just being a vegetarian—that it's about more than just being fit. I had become aware that we have to pay attention to *all* the risk factors if we're going to be following a comprehensive wellness program.

At that point, I had moved away from using egg yolks. I was avoiding dairy products in general, such as cheese and ice cream, which had been some of my favorite foods! I had given up these things cheerfully, because I knew I would be healthier. In the previous chapter, we talked about how important it is to set limits. The bottom line is that if we don't learn to set limits on our lives, our lives are going to set limits on us. We have to decide what is important to us. At that point in my life, I had decided that eating cheese and ice cream, as enjoyable as that was, was not as important as having a reasonable expectation of still being alive in twenty or thirty years to see my son and two daughters get married and have children of their own. I wanted to be able to play basketball with my kids. I wanted to be able to enjoy being with them and my grandchildren. I didn't want them to have to think about me like I had to think about my grandfather, whom I had never known.

My cholesterol levels were still running a little higher than I thought they should. So I decided to do a little project on myself. I had come a long way in the last six years. I was helping people reverse heart disease and improve their diabetes and do a lot of things to become healthier. I was more aware of my risks for heart disease. I was eating a much different diet than I had been six years earlier. *I wonder what would happen,* I thought, *if I went back a little toward the way I used to eat. I'll still eat a vegetarian diet, but it will be a lacto-ovo vegetarian diet. And I'll add a few food items I've taken off my list the last few years.*

So I started a three-week research project. Just three weeks. I added cheese and pizza to my diet. I enjoyed that. I added some ice cream as a dessert. I wasn't going crazy; I was eating my regular vegetarian diet but adding some other food to it. I started drinking milk.

Well, at the end of the first week, my overall cholesterol level went from 190 to 230. By the second week it was 257, and by the third week had risen to 280—after only twenty-one days of eating a vegetarian diet that included the saturated fat found in dairy, cheese, and ice cream. Yet most people would consider that a balanced diet. It was definitely a much better diet than the standard American diet.

Now I'm not saying this same result would happen to you. Everyone's metabolism is different, and you have to figure out what is going on in your own body. But the results were startling for me. I'm one of those persons whose standard lipid profile is enough to wave a big, red flag. My cholesterol and my triglycerides and my HDL and LDL—that was enough to make me stop and ask, "What's going on here? Something's wrong; I need to fix this."

For some of us, the 40 percent of risk factors for cardiovascular disease picked up by the standard lipid profile is enough to show us we have a problem. But for others of us, that's not enough. We need something to alert us to that other 60 percent of risk factors that increase our risk exponentially.

By the way, I went back to my earlier way of eating, and in three weeks my cholesterol level dropped 90 points! Some people are much more diet sensitive than others.

THE HUNTER HEART PROFILE

We can often begin to get a handle on the other 60 percent of risk factors for heart disease by doing an advanced cardiac profile such as the Hunter Heart Profile that I use in my clinic.

The first item on the Hunter Heart Profile is commonly referred to in the lipidology community as the "plaque test." It is FDA approved for assessing risk for both heart attacks and strokes. It tests for the lipoprotein phospholipase A2 enzyme, referred to on most lab panels as Lp-PLA2 and often referred to informally as the "PLAC test." This procedure actually measures whether you have active plaque in your artery walls. And it does so non-invasively. In certain situations it may still be necessary to actually go in invasively to see if there is plaque in the arteries, but the PLAC test can do that in most cases non-invasively. It also shows whether there's acute inflammation in the vascular bed, the inner lining of the artery wall.

> The presence of inflammation indicates that white blood cells are being attracted to that site, infiltrating the inner wall of the artery where they literally begin chewing up the toxic LDL cholesterol that has been oxidized, or turned rancid, in part because of the lack of adequate antioxidants in the diet.

That's why it is so important to make sure your diet contains whole foods that are loaded with antioxidant chemicals, fiber, and certain vitamins and nutrients.

Inadequate antioxidants in the diet allow the cholesterol to become oxidized, making it toxic to the artery wall. So the white blood cells, called *macrophages,* try to engulf this toxic cholesterol and chew it up to neutralize it. The word, *macrophage,* means "big eater." These white blood cells keep eating and sucking up all the toxic cholesterol until eventually they can't eat any more. What happens then? The white blood cells die. And that's what plaque is. It is thousands and thousands of dead white blood cells stuffed full of toxic cholesterol that has crystallized and turned into foam cells that you can actually squeeze together like Styrofoam. These foam cells are a gooey liquid similar to thick pus. This plaque inside the artery walls can rupture into the blood stream at any time and cause a clot to form almost instantly. Plaque is very, very damaging to the artery wall.

That's a tremendous risk for heart attacks and strokes. The whole idea is to try to prevent a clot which leads to a thrombus, completely plugging blood flow. If a thrombus forms in the carotid artery, the result is a loss of blood to the brain and possibly a stroke. If it forms in the coronary arteries, it can cause a heart attack. The problem in both cases is a loss of adequate blood supply. The brain or heart muscle that is deprived of blood will no longer receive the necessary oxygen or nutrients to those tissues—and they die. That's why circulation is so critical.

If the plaque test, the PLAC test, shows a result above 200, it means that there is active vascular inflammation or plaque buildup somewhere in the bloodstream. In that case, treatment needs to take place right away.

The PLAC test is an excellent test, especially in cases where a person is experiencing chest pain when they go outside and walk.

The second component of the Hunter Heart Profile is called the hs-CRP test, also referred to as the cardiac CRP. The acronym hs-CRP stands for High Sensitivity C-reactive Protein. The cardiac CRP tests for inflammation that influences the risk of heart disease that is not necessarily specific to the blood vessel wall. Results for the cardiac CRP can be high for a large number of reasons that may not involve plaque at all, at least not directly. For example, a person with rheumatoid arthritis or another autoimmune disease will tend to have a high cardiac CRP. However, this is still a very important test in assessing risk of heart disease. It is a much better predictor of heart disease than total cholesterol or LDL cholesterol levels.[2]

HDL, LDL, AND FIBER

Your body has some built-in ways of trying to deal with cholesterol and prevent its harmful effects on heart health. As you know, there is HDL cholesterol, the "good" cholesterol, and there is LDL cholesterol, the "bad" cholesterol. HDL works like a tow truck (some compare it to a garbage truck) to hook onto the LDL, the plaque-causing cholesterol, and take it to the liver which processes it and gets rid of it. Let's look a little more closely at how this works.

We saw earlier how LDL becomes toxic by being exposed to oxidizing agents, free radicals, and other toxins in the body. Then plaque is formed in the arteries as white blood cells die trying to engulf the toxic LDL. This leads to heart disease, strokes, and heart attacks. That's why the HDL, the "tow truck," tries to carry it to the liver for disposal.

But unless you are eating a natural, high-fiber diet, much of the work that the HDL does to move LDL to the liver for disposal is wasted. Without adequate fiber in your intestines, the LDL will simply be reabsorbed right back into your bloodstream. Here's why.

When the liver processes the toxic LDL, it dumps it into the gall bladder. At mealtimes, your gall bladder moves the LDL to your small intestine just in time to meet up with your food as it is leaving the stomach.

At that point, if there is abundant fiber in the food you have eaten, that fiber will literally grab hold of the toxic LDL and never let go. The LDL is eliminated in your next bowel movement. But that can't happen without fiber in your diet. Without sufficient fiber, you're missing the opportunity to get rid of that toxic cholesterol. You're also missing the opportunity to decrease inflammatory stress on every organ system in the body—the brain, the heart, the kidneys, the eyes, every organ.

THE HDL PARADOX

But there is an interesting paradox about HDL cholesterol—the good cholesterol. On average, having a higher HDL *lowers* your risk of cardiovascular or coronary heart disease.[3] In other words, the higher the HDL cholesterol, the better, right? Well, that's where statistics kind of get in the way of reality. The higher the better when it comes to HDL is technically true, but it doesn't necessarily apply to you or me.

For instance, I already mentioned that when I added dairy and pizza and ice cream to my vegetarian diet for three weeks a number of years ago, my total cholesterol went from 190 to 280. But my HDL nearly doubled in those three weeks! That should be a positive thing if it's true that the higher one's HDL, the lower the risk of heart disease. But studies have now demonstrated that for some individuals, very high HDL levels actually represent higher risk for active heart disease.[4] For these persons, cardiovascular atherosclerosis is more active with higher HDL levels.

Another way to look at this paradox is that having a high HDL means you have a whole bunch of cholesterol tow trucks trying to move toxic LDL cholesterol from the arteries to the liver. But what does that tell you?

What does that mean? A lot of tow trucks must mean that you have a lot of dysfunctional, broken-down vehicles that need hauling away. A lot of toxic LDL that needs to be towed to the liver. And that's not good.

Another way to understand this paradox is the analogy of how your body responds to infection with a fever. Is fever a good thing? Well, nobody likes to have a fever because it doesn't feel good. But what would happen to us if an infection *didn't* cause us to have a fever? Without fever, our immune system would not be mobilized nearly as effectively as it might be. And that means we could die from a simple infection just because the body wasn't able to mobilize an aggressive inflammatory response against that virus or bacteria or whatever was causing the infection. So fever is a good thing—as long as you're managing it and it eventually does its job of eradicating the infection.

It's the same with HDL. HDL is a good thing—as long as you're managing it and it eventually does its job. The problem with a chronically elevated HDL is that it suggests you are chronically toxic and chronically inflamed. If so, you need to find out what is really going on inside your body. Fortunately, we have some advanced cardiac risk tools involving lifestyle and nutritional medicine to help us understand that, evaluate it properly, and then act on it aggressively. That's the first step. There are medications, too, that can help manage those problems. Your goal, and that of your doctor, should be to figure out as much as possible, how you can control your risk factors naturally. There is plenty of research going on today that gives us information on how to do just that.

Ironically, some of the populations in the world that have the lowest documented rates of heart disease also have the lowest HDL levels anywhere. Certain Japanese populations and the Tarahumara Indians in southern Mexico are well-known for very low cardiovascular risk, yet they have HDL levels that, by American standards, are an independent risk factor for heart disease. In reality, as a people, they have one of the lowest risks for heart disease in the world.[5]

So it's a real paradox. What I'm suggesting is that you can't just flippantly look at your lipid risk factors and say, "My cholesterol levels are good. Yes, my overall cholesterol may be a little high, but my HDL is high enough that the ratio looks good. So I'm okay."

Maybe it is good that your HDL is high, but it could also be that it's high because it's indicating a problem. You need to consider that possibility.

CIRCULATION AND INFLAMMATION

We've known about the link between inflammation and heart disease for some time. In 2004, *Time* magazine published a cover story pointing out the connection between inflammation and heart attacks, cancer, Alzheimer's, and other diseases. The article also gave some suggestions on what you can do to address inflammation. That was pretty proactive for a general interest magazine. Yet years later, we're still trying to incorporate the things we know to do about inflammation into the typical clinical practice, because almost all our efforts are still focused on blood pressure and cholesterol, even though they don't represent the majority of the risk for heart disease.

Dr. Paul Ridker, a cardiologist at Harvard, did a study[6] showing that as one's cardiac CRP, the measure of inflammation, gradually increases, it dramatically increases the risk of having a heart attack or stroke. He divided the test population into five equal groups based on cardiac CRP levels. Those with the lowest risk of having a subsequent heart attack had a cardiac CRP level, a measure of systemic inflammation, that was less than 0.6. The optimal level is actually 0.35, so the lower the inflammation, the better. I believe everyone should have this cardiac CRP inflammation test, because it is twice as predictive of having a cardiovascular event as is the standard cholesterol test.

If your cardiac CRP level reaches 2.0, that means 60 percent of Americans have a level of inflammation that is lower than yours.[7] If your level is higher than 2.0, it means that the great majority of Americans are doing better with inflammation than you are. Again, you don't ever want to be in a position on anything where the majority of people in America have a lower risk than you do.

What if you score high on *these two* components of the Hunter Heart Profile—the cardiac CRP test and the PLAC test? Let's say your PLAC test is above 200 and your cardiac CRP is above 2.0. In that case, you are facing an eleven-fold[8] greater risk for stroke!

But even in that case, you don't have to give up. You don't have to sit back and say, "I guess I don't have a chance."

Yes, you do! You still have a huge opportunity to enjoy health and wellness. You see, even bad news is valuable. Knowing your statistical risk means that you and your doctor can immediately intervene and that you have a better knowledge of just exactly what needs to be done. Awareness is a call to action. Medical science today is helping us to know just how to reverse specific risks. So there is much that you can do.

REVERSING HEART DISEASE

Some twenty years ago, I had the opportunity to meet Dr. James Barnard of the UCLA School of Medicine. Dr. Barnard was the person who worked closely with Nathan Pritikin, the engineer who in the 1970s figured out on his own how to reverse heart disease. It all started when two of the most prominent cardiologists in Los Angeles told Pritikin that there was nothing they could do for him.

"Are you serious?" he asked them. "You went through years of medical training just to tell me that you can't do anything about my heart disease?"

"Mr. Pritikin," they explained, "you need to understand that you have more than 90 percent occlusion in multiple blood vessels of the heart. It's been demonstrated for decades that when heart disease progresses this far, it's completely irreversible. It can't be fixed."

You should never tell an engineer that something can't be fixed! Engineers know that *anything* is fixable. With enough time and money, they can figure out how to solve any problem. Nathan Pritikin said, "You're obviously not interested in fixing my heart disease, so I'll figure it out for myself."

He started spending more than twenty hours every week at the UCLA library examining the research relating to the possibility of reversing heart disease. He couldn't find much research dealing with humans, but he found tons of research on animals. He found a lot of studies on reversing heart disease in animals. Now, Pritikin knew that animals aren't humans, but he figured that the circulation systems and the risk factors for heart disease must be essentially the same for both. So he started applying the knowledge he gained from the medical research done on animals, research that had been in the files for decades. Within weeks he had reversed his unstable angina. He had no more chest pain. Within a few months, all his cardiac risk factors had returned to normal, and he was fully functional.

Before he died of an unrelated illness more than two decades later, Nathan Pritikin told a cardiologist friend, "I want you to be at my autopsy, and I want you to write an editorial and print it in a medical journal showing what happened to my heart after changing my diet and lifestyle."

He had reversed his heart disease. It was reported that, at his death, Nathan Pritikin had the arteries of a teenager, not the occluded arteries of a man who had once been given just weeks to live but who ended up living decades longer.

ADDRESSING THE HEALTH FACTORS WITHOUT MEDICATION

Dr. James Barnard, who had worked intimately with Nathan Pritikin, published an interesting study in 2004. This study followed a group of women for just three weeks in a comprehensive wellness program in which they didn't just exercise, and they didn't just eat an optimal, plant-based diet—they did everything that was known to be part of a healing cardiac program. Dr. Bernard was able to document that in just three weeks their level of inflammation in their blood, their cardiac CRP, dropped 40 percent.[9] It plummeted. Far more than if they'd gone on the medications usually prescribed for lowering inflammation. Far more than if they'd been taking the statin medications that lower cholesterol and inflammation about 30 percent. When you apply a comprehensive approach, you get dramatic, comprehensive transformation.

About this same time, at the clinic where I did lifestyle medicine in Guam, we had been demonstrating month after month that by putting individuals on a comprehensive program including a plant-based diet, appropriate supplements, daily exercise, and carefully managing all risk factors, we were able to lower cardiac CRP inflammation levels by an average of 50 percent in just two weeks.

Dr. Paul Ridker, the Harvard cardiologist who was one of the first to promote using the cardiac CRP test, had published a study showing that people with high inflammation levels were at high risk of heart disease even if their cholesterol levels were normal. The study began with about 18,000 people and was supposed to continue for four or five years.

Dr. Ridker put one group of individuals on a statin cholesterol-lowering medication, even though their cholesterol levels were normal. After a year to eighteen months, these individuals had lowered their risk of a heart attack by 44 percent!

Why? They didn't need to lower their cholesterol, so why did the cholesterol-lowering medication reduce their cardiac risk so dramatically? Dr. Ridker found that it was because the medication also lowered their inflammation levels by over 30 percent.[10]

I wanted to read Dr. Ridker's study more carefully. This was some years ago, and buying a copy on the Internet would cost me twenty-five dollars. But I knew that in the research community, if I sent the author an email requesting a copy, he had the right to send me one free—and that he probably would. So I sent Dr. Ridker an email saying how much I would appreciate a copy of the study for further review. Then I added that in the wellness programs conducted in my clinic we had been able to reduce cardiac CRP by 50 percent in just two weeks using a comprehensive lifestyle program and diet.

I expected his graduate assistant to send me a copy of the study saying, "We're pleased to send this to you; have a nice day." But a couple of days later, I received an email from Dr. Ridker himself. He sent me the study, but he wrote, "I am very intrigued by your work, because I fully believe that nothing is more powerful in lowering inflammation in the body, the type of inflammation that causes premature disease and death, than an optimal diet."

This was the person doing all the *drug* research. Why would he say that diet is the most powerful factor in lowering inflammation? Because anyone who has done research in these areas has to study the big picture. They have to study it broadly to properly understand what all the research shows on that topic, and they all know what the most powerful strategies are for decreasing risk.

In the previous chapter we learned that daily, moderate exercise can lower inflammation in our body substantially.[11] Drinking enough water is also important in dealing with systemic inflammation. Make sure you are drinking enough water throughout the day. You should take in at least eight ounces of water , preferably sixteen ounces, at the very start of the day. Why? Because you're dehydrated from losing water all night through breathing, perspiration, and creating urine. So it's important to rehydrate when you wake up at the beginning of the day. If you don't, you're at a higher risk of developing a clot.

One of the easiest and most important ways to lower your risk of having a clot or a cardiovascular problem is to make sure to rehydrate yourself with pure, filtered water each morning when you wake up.

If you have any tendency to constipation, make that warm to hot water. Do this a few days in a row, within ten to fifteen minutes of waking up, and you will have a full elimination. It is also help you lower your risk of toxicities that cause inflammation.

One interesting finding, even in the drug studies that look at lowering cardiac risk or the amount of plaque buildup in the arterial walls, is that simply adding a nutrient, such as niacin or Vitamin B3, or an essential oil such as EPA or DHA, can often almost double the benefit that a regular medication would have.[12] These studies are now suggesting that there are many things we can do to dramatically improve our cardiac risk without having to jump on the medication bandwagon.

We know that the more fit an individual is, on average, the lower will be his or her cardiac CRP level as a measure of inflammation. Being fit cuts inflammation by more than half compared to being unfit.[13] So even though fitness doesn't in and of itself make you healthy, as we pointed out in Chapter 2, it does powerfully alter and mitigate risk in general. It's important to pay attention to fitness and include it in your overall health and wellness program.

THE FOODS MOST LIKELY TO CAUSE INFLAMMATION

Many researchers are saying that cardiac disease, atherosclerosis, is basically an inflammatory disease. It isn't just a matter of clogged plumbing. It is an actual inflammatory condition and that to deal with it we must learn how to lower inflammation.

> The studies continue to show that the gradual buildup of oxidized LDL cholesterol in the artery wall, especially when combined with inflammation, leads to vulnerable plaque—plaque that is just waiting to create a cardiac problem.

As plaque forms it's possible to observe the thickening of the inner arterial wall. The dead, white blood cells are oozing toxic cholesterol, ready to form a clot. The release of enzymes from the plaque-infected artery wall can be easily detected by the PLAC test.

Harvard did a great study a few years ago. After all this information about inflammation became apparent, researchers at Harvard said, "Hey! We have frozen blood samples that have been collected every few years for the past thirty years. We can go back to thirty years of these samples and measure this new cardiac CRP blood test."

So they did. They examined frozen blood samples collected as early as 1976 from more than 100,000 doctors and nurses. From that data they were able to show, based on careful dietary histories of the participants, which food were most responsible for causing inflammation.[14]

1. Processed meats. The Harvard study found that one of the foods most associated with an elevated cardiac CRP was processed meats.[15] Processed meats dramatically increase the risk of diabetes. Inflammation turns on the diabetes genes. Processed meats dramatically increase the risk of heart disease, because they are inflammatory and inflammation turns on the genes that promote heart disease. The list of problems connected to processed meats because of increased inflammation goes on and on and on. An additional reason is that processed meats are more likely than other meat products to contain toxins.

There is a great deal of concern today about pesticides found in fruits and vegetables. And don't misunderstand; that is an important concern. It is great when people decide to go completely organic. But the amount of pesticides and toxins found in just one serving of animal products far outweighs the amount of toxins you would ingest after days and days of consuming vegetables and fruits that have been sprayed with pesticides. Why? Because animals concentrate toxins. We humans concentrate toxins. So when we consume the flesh of an animal that has been concentrating toxins during its entire life, we're being exposed to a lot of toxicity.

Toxicity is one of the main reasons processed meats increase inflammation so drastically and thus increase risk factors for cardiac disease. Processed meats often include organ meats, which are likely to contain the most toxins and heavy metals. Organ meats are also most likely to be infectious. What do infections do? They increase inflammation. Do you see how all these pieces fit together?

2. *Refined grains.* You can be completely vegan and have a very inflammation-prone diet. A lot of unhealthy things are vegan. So the focus isn't whether you're a vegan or a vegetarian. The focus should be on determining the most healthful diet. You need to be focused on first-class foods—foods that are known to improve health. And what are those foods? What does the scientific evidence show? Plant-based whole foods. That's the most important consideration. Make sure you are getting plenty of plant-based, whole foods in your diet.

3. *Refined sweets.* Pastries, cakes, cookies, candy, pies, etc. We all know that we need to be careful to limit these kinds of things, right? It's a no brainer. They are high calorie, highly refined, non-nutritious—and very good at increasing inflammation in the body.

4. *Diet sodas.* This fourth category isn't really a food group at all. Many people think they are doing their body a favor by drinking a diet soda instead of one filled with sugar. That is not necessarily true. You might wonder how something that has no caloric value whatsoever can cause inflammation. Well, arsenic, lead, mercury, pesticides, and all kinds of toxins have no caloric value whatsoever either. But they certainly cause inflammation and neurotoxicity.

A new study presented recently at meetings of the American College of Cardiology looked at a subset from about 60,000 women who had been involved a study called the Women's Health Initiative.

In the new study, Dr. Vyas, of the University of Iowa, found that women who consumed diet sodas on a regular basis—defined as two per day—had a 30 percent increased risk of having a heart attack compared to women who rarely or never drank diet sodas.

> Now many people would think that drinking two diet sodas a day was no big deal. After all, they don't have any calories, so why not? But the study found this significantly increased risk of a heart attack. It also found that drinking two diet sodas a day increased the risk of premature death by 50 percent! This was a huge epidemiological study that lasted about nine years.

Other studies indicate that even for weight loss diet soda isn't helpful. The evidence seems to be that people who drink diet sodas regularly are more likely to gain weight—even compared to those who drink regular sodas. That's puzzling, because regular soda is loaded with calories. But regardless of calories or no calories, the big issue is inflammation. I'm not saying calories aren't important; I'm saying calories are much less important than inflammation.

STICKY CHOLESTEROL

There are other blood tests that are valuable for assessing cardiac risk. One of these looks at lipoprotein (a), also known as the "sticky LDL cholesterol." Sticky cholesterol is related to a genetic mutation. If you have elevated levels of sticky cholesterol—30 or higher—that represents an increased risk of heart disease. The amount of plaque-forming cholesterol contained in sticky cholesterol is ten times greater than regular LDL cholesterol.[16] So it's important to know your sticky cholesterol level. There are some specific nutritional strategies that work to lower this risk factor.

SMALL, DENSE LDL (SD-LDL)

LDL is the "bad" cholesterol, but a variant of LDL is even worse. Small, dense LDL (sd-LDL) is an LDL particle that is so small it can easily infiltrate the artery wall and cause plaque. So if it is determined that your levels of sd-LDL are elevated, you can't just take statin medications as a way of combating it. In fact, some of the statin cholesterol-lowering medications actually increase the sticky cholesterol and small, dense cholesterol.

FOCUSING ON THE BIG PICTURE

It is so critical that we focus first on the big picture. Remember the crucial importance of the exposome—all the things in our lives that influence our risks for some type of serious health problem. As we test for different risk factors, our knowledge of the big picture becomes clearer. We begin to have insight into what we can do, not just to manage risk, but to actually *reverse* risk!

So, again, I want to suggest that, as you become more knowledgeable about what needs to be included in your personal wellness program, you become serious about setting limits in your life and making choices that will lead to better health and a richer, fuller life.

In health, as in every area of life, you have to decide what is most important to you, and then develop a plan that will enable you to reach those priorities. By definition, that plan is going to include things that you *should* do, and it must, by definition, also include things that you're *not* going to do. Those are the two keys of strategic planning that dramatically increase your chances of succeeding in your wellness program.

Remember, you are in charge of your health; no one else can take on that role for you.

CHAPTER SUMMARY

>> You can't have good health without good circulation.

>> Exercise causes the muscles to act like mini-pumps, helping the heart move blood around the body.

>> A traditional lipid profile addresses only about 40 percent of the risk factors for a heart attack or stroke.

>> Wellness means more than simply being fit.

>> Advanced cardiac lab tests such as the Hunter Heart Profile helps identify the 60 percent of risk factors for heart attack and stroke not addressed by the traditional lipid profile.

>> There is a definite link between systemic inflammation and cardiac disease.

>> Heart disease can be reversed.

>> A comprehensive wellness program including a plant-based diet, daily exercise, and appropriate supplements can result in dramatically reducing inflammation and risk factors for cardiac disease.

>> Processed meats, refined grains, refined sweets, and diet sodas are the main dietary culprits in causing increased systemic inflammation.

ENDNOTES

1   Ridker, P., "Proposed Cardiovascular Risk Assessment Algorithm Using High-Sensitivity C-Reactive Protein and Lipid Screening," *Clinical Chemistry,* January 2001, vol. 47, no. 1; 28-30.

2   Ibid.

3   Executive Summary of the Third Report of the National Cholesterol Education Program (NCEP) Expert Panel on Detection, Evaluation, and Treatment of High Blood Cholesterol in Adults (Adult Treatment Panel III). *JAMA.* May 16, 2001; 285(19): 2486-2497.

4   Vibhuti, N. Singh, M.D., "High HDL Cholesterol (Hyperalphalipoproteinemia)," *Medscape.* Updated December 18, 2014.

5   McMurry, M. P.; Cerqueira, M. T.; Connor, S. L.; Connor, W. E., "Changes in Lipid and Lipoprotein Levels and Body Weight in Tarahumarn Indians After Consumption of an Affluent Diet," *New England Journal of Medicine,* 1991; 325:1754–1758.

6   Ridker, P. M., et al., *New England Journal of Medicine,* 2002; 347:1557-1565.

7   http://lipidsonline.org/commentaries/cme_pdf/commentary_037.pdf

8 Ballantyne, C. M.; Hoogeveen, R. C.; Bang, H.; et al., "Lipoprotein-Associated Phospholipase A2, High-Sensitivity C-Reactive Protein, and Risk for Incident Ischemic Stroke in Middle-Aged Men and Women in the Atherosclerosis Risk in Communities (ARIC) Study," *Arch Intern Med,* November 28, 2005, 165(21):2479-2484.

9 Wegge, J; Barnard, J; "Effect of Diet and Exercise Intervention on Inflammatory and Adhesion Molecules in Postmenopausal Women on Hormone Replacement Therapy and at Risk for Coronary Artery Disease," *Metabolism—Clinical and Experimental,* vol. 53, issue 3, 377-381.

10 Ridker, P., "Rosuvastatin to Prevent Vascular Events in Men and Women with Elevated C-Reactive Protein," *New England Journal of Medicine,* 2008, 359:2195-2207.

11 Church, T. S., et al., "Associations Between Cardiorespiratory Fitness and C-Reactive Protein in Men," *Arteriosclerosis, Thrombosis, and Vascular Biology,* November, 1, 2002; 22:1869-1876.

12 "Optimizing Patient Cardiovascular Care with the Hunter Heart Profile," a 2014 presentation by Paul Ziajka, M.D., Ph.D., Director of The Florida Lipid Institute; Diplomat of the American Board of Clinical Lipidology; President of the South East Lipid Association.

13 Church, T. S., et al., "Associations Between Cardiorespiratory Fitness and C-Reactive Protein in Men," *Arteriosclerosis, Thrombosis, and Vascular Biology,* November, 1, 2002; 22:1869-1876.

14 Giugliano, D., "The Effects of Diet on Inflammation: Emphasis on the Metabolic Syndrome," *Journal of the American College of Cardiology,* vol. 48, issue 4, August 15, 2006, pp. 677–685.

15 Ley, S. H.; Sun, Q.; Willett, W. C.; et al., "Associations Between Red Meat Intake and Biomarkers of Inflammation and Glucose Metabolism in Women," *American Journal of Clinical Nutrition,* 2014; 99:352-360.

16 "Optimizing Patient Cardiovascular Care with the Hunter Heart Profile," a 2014 presentation by Paul Ziajka, M.D., Ph.D., Director of The Florida Lipid Institute; Diplomat of the American Board of Clinical Lipidology; President of the South East Lipid Association.

FOUR

Here Comes the Sun!

SUNLIGHT, VITAMIN D AND HEALTH

IN THIS CHAPTER I'M GOING TO TELL YOU ABOUT a miracle drug. This awesome, miracle drug kills bacteria powerfully. It does this by stimulating the DNA within the nucleus of every cell to provide a special code that the cell then uses to manufacture cathelicidin, a protein antimicrobial peptide, that the body's immune system utilizes to destroy viruses and cancers and bacteria—anything that isn't supposed to be in the body.

The body's immune system is designed to protect it from disease-causing entities. It's like an army whose mission it is to fight off anything that threatens the body's wellbeing. But like any other army, the immune system needs ammunition. An army without ammunition isn't going to be able to achieve very much. That's why the immune system must have this antimicrobial peptide, a germ-killing protein, in order to successfully attack the things it needs to destroy.

This miracle drug I'm talking about stimulates the production of the immune system's ammunition—antimicrobial peptide. It's one of the best ways to kill bacteria. This miracle drug will greatly protect you against pneumonia. It fights tuberculosis. In fact, if used properly, this drug could potentially eradicate tuberculosis completely. It can add years to your life; it can synchronize hormones; it can beautify skin; it protects against sixteen different types of cancer; it protects against multiple sclerosis; it fights binge eating, it drives away depression, and it helps prevent falls in the elderly, lowering risk of hip fractures dramatically. It increases agility and makes the muscles stronger. It helps prevents chronic kidney failure. In fact, it can even reverse Stage 3, and potentially Stage 4, chronic kidney failure.[1]

At this point, you're probably thinking, *What is this guy trying to sell me? How much is this going to cost?*

I'm not selling anything. But if such a miracle drug were available—one that would be able to provide all these health benefits—how much would you be willing to pay for it?

PURE, SIMPLE SUNLIGHT

The good news is that there is such a "drug," and it's free! I'm talking about sunlight. Pure, simple, sunlight contains many properties—including the production of Vitamin D—that can actually bring about all these benefits I've listed and tremendously increase your health and wellness.

> Ever since the early 1980s, we have heard a media blitz concerning how bad sunlight is. I would like to try to change that tide of negative opinion.

For a great many of us, sunlight is a wellness strategy that is missing and therefore limiting us in our goal of achieving our full genetic potential. In fact, if you're not taking advantage of the benefits of sunlight, it could be one reason why everything else you're doing to maximize your health isn't really helping as much as it could.

VITAMIN D DEFICIENCY

Let me share with you a study regarding Vitamin D. In 2009, at a large conference of the American Medical Association, researchers presented the results of a study on the levels of Vitamin D in teenagers and how those levels dramatically affect their risk for disease. They divided the subjects of the study into four groups based on the level of Vitamin D in their blood. Then they compared the group with the lowest levels—less than 15 nanograms per milliliter (ng/mL)[2]—with the group having the highest levels of Vitamin D. What they found was fascinating.

Those who had the lowest levels of Vitamin D were 2.3 times more likely to have high blood pressure than those in the group with the highest levels.

Their risk of having high blood sugar, or prediabetes, was 2.5 times greater. Their risk of metabolic syndrome, or insulin resistance—which is known to be the number one risk factor for heart attacks and strokes as we age—was increased almost four times because of their low levels of Vitamin D.[3]

Here is the sobering part of this study. As the researchers looked at the spectrum of teenagers in the study, they found that the average Vitamin D blood levels varied somewhat by race. For white teenagers it was 28 ng/mL, for Hispanics, 21.5, and for black youth, 15. But the important finding was this: teenagers of all races were Vitamin D deficient. Yes, Hispanics and whites had slightly higher levels of Vitamin D, but not enough to be considered adequate. In reality, all three groups were deficient in this important nutrient. In other words, insufficient Vitamin D is a problem for nearly all of us.

When a patient has his or her Vitamin D blood level tested, the lab report typically suggests a normal reference range of 30 to 100 ng/mL. Levels less than 30 are considered to be inadequate.

When I first learned about the connection between low Vitamin D levels and many diseases, I began testing every patient. While living on the sunny, Pacific island of Guam, I was shocked that most of my patients had low levels of Vitamin D when tested. I soon learned that Vitamin D deficiency is everywhere—even in areas where least expected. And the problem seems to be getting worse each year. Between 1988 and 2004, the rate of Vitamin D deficiency in the United States skyrocketed from 55 to 77 percent.[4]

My good friend, Eric Madrid, M.D., wrote a book, *The Vitamin D Prescription: The Healing Power of the Sun & How It Can Save Your Life.*[5] As part of his research, Dr. Madrid tested all the patients in his Southern California family practice clinic. Reporting on his findings, Dr. Madrid explained to me, "Eighty percent of my patients had Vitamin D levels below 32, while 90 percent of my senior and African American populations were low."

One of the biggest challenges for doctors who prescribe statin cholesterol-lowering medications is that at least 20 percent of the patients for whom they prescribe these medications develop joint and muscle pain. I'm not talking about just a little pain; I'm talking about significant pain—pain that causes them to have to discontinue the medication within a couple of weeks. When this happens, their physician will often refer them to a lipidologist—a physician specializing in disorders of cholesterol and blood lipids. One lipidologist recently stated that 95 percent of the patients who are referred to him because they are not tolerating statin medications, are unable to do so because they are Vitamin D deficient.[6]

IS VITAMIN D REALLY IMPORTANT?

I should also mention that several large studies published in the spring of 2014 have cast doubt on the whole concept of Vitamin D being a valuable nutrient. After conducting studies and crunching numbers, these researches have concluded that we really ought to be backing away from the idea of recommending Vitamin D supplements. In fact, they conclude that we probably don't need to be measuring Vitamin D levels at all.

I could not disagree more with those conclusions. Sunlight and Vitamin D constitute a critical piece of the wellness package that you should be paying attention to.

> If you follow health issues with any degree of interest at all, you know that there are a lot of different opinions on every topic. In fact, there are many different studies on every topic, and it's possible to pick and choose the studies that fit your perspective.

But the true seeker for health will follow the evidence, searching out what is really important for general public health, but even more importantly, what works for himself or herself in the quest for individual wellness.

I have had the privilege of talking with four of the world's leading experts in Vitamin D in clinical practice. I have had the privilege of attending three international conferences on Vitamin D. It's a fascinating topic, because so many people are ignoring the role of Vitamin D in their health. It's a missing element. They are not only ignoring Vitamin D, they are trying to avoid it, because of all the negative information about sunlight and Vitamin D.

That is why I feel this issue must be addressed. When you read or hear of a new study that seems to cast doubt on the idea of using sunlight healthfully and optimizing Vitamin D blood levels, you might ask, "Should I follow the conclusions of this study or should I look to experts who have been studying this subject for fifty years or more? Experts who haven't conducted just a single study or statistical analysis, but who have actually been thinking about it and studying it and asking the right questions for many, many decades?"

Whose conclusions are you going to believe? It doesn't matter what organization has conducted the study. What matters is whether the research is credible given all the evidence.

I mentioned that lipidologists are finding that the great majority of individuals who are unable to tolerate statin cholesterol-lowering medications due to pain are Vitamin D deficient. They are also finding that most of those unable to tolerate statin medication can do so once their Vitamin D blood levels are adequate. That fact alone, given recent recommendations about the importance of lowering cholesterol, should be enough to do away with the notion of no longer testing and optimizing Vitamin D blood levels.

The importance of Vitamin D in the context of cholesterol and cardiovascular risk is highlighted as well by the fact that those taking a statin medication to lower cholesterol experience some degree of muscle damage as a result of the medication.

They may not have joint or muscle pain, but muscle biopsies studies have shown that there is microscopic muscle damage present.[7] Furthermore, it has been shown that more than half of individuals who actually develop muscle or joint pain after starting cholesterol medication also had a more significant level of muscle cell damage classified as muscle injury.[8] This ought to tell us that we should be paying attention to the role of Vitamin D as a wellness factor that is critical to our health.

SUNLIGHT AND CARDIOVASCULAR HEALTH

Do you know what time of day you are most likely to suffer a heart attack? The answer is: early in the morning, right around the time that you wake up. During that first hour after waking is when our bodies are most at risk, physiologically, psychologically, and emotionally, of succumbing to a heart attack. The chance of having a heart attack first thing in the morning is significantly greater than the potential for having one at another time.[9]

Why is that? A couple of hours before we wake up, the body begins to produce and release cortisol, a stress hormone. It's supposed to be released gradually so that when we wake up, we feel good. The problem is that cortisol also increases clotting, which in turn increases blood pressure. All this makes it more likely for any atherosclerotic plaque in the coronary arteries to break open, plugging the artery and causing a heart attack.

So, what are some things you could be doing right now, some things you could begin putting into practice tomorrow morning, to dramatically reduce your personal risk of having a cardiovascular event—a heart attack?

I would suggest that one of the most wonderful gifts that you have available to you—and a way to reduce your cardiac risk—is the opportunity to enjoy the early morning light outdoors. Drink a large glass of water, first thing in the morning. Go outside in the sunshine.

A little walk adds to the benefit, but even just sitting outside in the morning sunshine will make a powerful change, psychologically and physiologically, in the way you approach the day.

SYNCHRONIZING YOUR BIOLOGICAL CLOCK

We humans have a biological clock that synchronizes with the cycle of light and darkness. We need to spend an optimal amount of time outside in the light. The research suggests anywhere from thirty to sixty minutes of sunshine. I'm not talking about spending two hours out in the sun in the heat of the day. I'm talking about up to an hour of exposure to sunshine in the early morning or late afternoon. Exposure to outside light during the day helps your pineal gland to release much-needed melatonin at night. Melatonin is a restorative hormone that helps your body heal. It also promotes sleep. If you cannot sleep well, your body isn't able to restore or rejuvenate itself well. You are at risk of speeding up the aging process and making the body more receptive to disease.

> You want to speed the healing process, and that requires good sleep which requires time outdoors exposed to the light. Based on the research, morning—especially early morning in the first few hours after sunrise—is the best time to be out in the sunshine.[10] And it not only promotes physical wellness, it does wonders for you psychologically as well.

In 1988, I was given an opportunity to go to Singapore for the summer to do a lifestyle medicine internship at Youngberg Memorial Hospital, named after my great uncle. He had been one of the first Christian missionaries to the island of Borneo in the early 1930s. I flew from Los Angeles to Seoul, Korea, and then on to Singapore. I arrived late at night after flying for almost twenty-four hours. My biological clock was completely off!

I went from the airport to the hospital, where I met the president of the institution. He said to me, "By the way, we are doing a 5K run tomorrow morning right across from the hospital. Would you like to take part?"

I cringed inside, because morning was only a few hours away, and I was so tired. But I smiled and replied, "Of course. I'd love to do that." I didn't want to make a bad first impression as a lifestyle medicine intern.

The president offered to wake me for the run. Sure enough, at 5:00 o'clock in the morning, he was knocking on my door. I crawled out of bed and tried to look energetic. A little later, I found myself running the 5K in Singapore's "100 percent" humidity. All I could think of was, "I'm going to die!" My chest was ready to explode, and I was trying to make it look easy, because I was the "wellness guy." I smiled and just sucked up the pain and discomfort. After that

5K, I was exhausted. But something really strange happened. I was expecting to experience at least two or three days of jet lag. But that early morning run, in the bright morning light, completely reset my circadian rhythm. I had no jet lag at all.

The lesson for you? If you travel by air across several time zones and are expecting to have jet lag, get up early according to the local time at your destination. Expose yourself to the bright morning light along with a little exercise that causes you to breathe deeply. You'll find your jet lag is diminished dramatically.

Even when you're home and following your normal routine, you need to pay attention to your internal clock and synchronize it appropriately. When you go outside in the early morning light, you're re-syncing your clock and improving your ability to restore your health throughout the next 24-hour cycle. A whole new field of medicine, called chronobiology, is involved in paying attention to the importance of timing. There are times that are best for all our activities—exercise, eating, going to bed, waking up. For example, chronobiology is finding that it's not just how long you sleep that's important, but how smart you sleep. And timing is a major part of that.

SUNLIGHT AND WEIGHT CONTROL

Can sunlight actually help with weight control?

Animal studies have shown that exposure to early morning sunshine can result in weight loss—without making any change at all to the animals' caloric intake.[11]

> Calories are important, of course, but I'm suggesting that there are many other variables that are critical components of weight control—variables that regulate our hormones and our metabolism, things that regulate how we feel emotionally and psychologically, as well as physically.

I have two dogs, and I like to take them to the dog park once in a while. If you've done that, have you noticed what often happens? While the dogs are off running around and having a good time, what are their human owners doing? Sitting on the park bench in the shade. We should be taking advantage of the sunlight and getting activity as well.

Recently published studies show that obese women, exposed to sunlight for at least forty-five minutes between the hours of 6:00 and 9:00 A.M., actually begin losing weight after a couple of weeks.[12]

Now, researchers often try to isolate different variables in order to determine which one has the greatest impact on a given finding. So in these studies, they controlled for caloric intake, trying to determine if sunlight is actually beneficial in terms of weight loss. But it's often difficult to say with certainty if a particular factor is the most important factor or whether it is more important than some other component. As I have worked over the years with strategies for increasing wellness, I have learned that when a person takes advantage of a new wellness strategy and adds it to his or her lifestyle, that new strategy makes all the other positive things he or she is doing even more effective. For example, as you get the psychological benefit of being exposed to sunlight, your craving for carbohydrates goes way down. So what happens then? Your tendency to binge on a given food, especially foods that are not good for you, diminishes dramatically.

So I believe that in terms of weight control, the issue isn't whether sunlight is more important than restricting calories. The important issue is to be sure you are taking advantage of *all* the missing elements in your life so that everything works the way it should to increase your health and wellness.

Other studies have shown that for sleep-deprived individuals, just a couple of hours of exposure to sunlight will actually rebalance the leptin and ghrelin hormones that determine feelings of fullness from eating a meal.[13] If you are not sleeping well, partly because you are not exposed to early morning sunlight, the hormones that should make you feel satisfied after eating, don't work well. You've developed a resistance to the satisfaction hormones. Your body doesn't feel satisfied after eating a sufficient amount. The solution is to try to care for all the deficiencies in your life that cause poor health.

SUNLIGHT AND MELANOMA

"Alright," some may say. "Maybe sunlight has some real benefits to offer, but what about the other side of the story? What if I feel better now, but in ten years I develop melanoma from all this exposure to sunlight? Could the treatment be worse than the cure?"

Let's look at the research.

Studies show that regular exposure to prudent amounts of sunshine actually protects against lymphoma and melanoma.[14, 15] For example, studies at the Karolinsk Institute have demonstrated that sunshine exposure cuts the risk of non-Hodgkins lymphoma up to 40 percent and protects against other cancers as well.[16] In 2005, the *Journal of the National Cancer Institute* published a study showing that exposure to sunlight actually was linked with better survival rates in people with melanoma.[17]

My reading and experience in this area tell me that we need to be paying attention to the big picture. We need to be asking, "What is really best from a holistic health standpoint?" The very thing that people are avoiding could be critical to reaching their wellness potential; we need to reason from cause to effect in these matters.

Based on research, sun-related melanomas are much less aggressive than other types of melanomas, such as those related to diet. What does diet have to do with melanoma skin cancer? Personally, I believe diet has a lot to do with melanoma. I believe a large number of melanomas are actually caused by diet.

How could that be?

Consider the typical slaughter house scenario. A cow, for example, that is being slaughtered has a visible melanoma. That animal is immediately taken off the line and the entire animal is incinerated—right? Absolutely not! At best, the obvious melanoma is cut out, and the rest of the animal is sent on down the meat-packing line. Do you think cutting out the obviously diseased area removes most of the melanoma? Melanoma is often systemic. What happens when a person eats the meat from that cow?

In many cases the disease still present in that meat won't necessarily be taken care of by digestion. Diseases, and even portions of cancerous tissues, in what we eat could be transferred intact into the bloodstream. This isn't something that you will hear much about. But I believe it is one of the reasons that processed meats are so high on the list of food groups associated with inflammation. That is why I strongly recommend staying away from processed meats.

What about processed vegetarian meat substitutes?

It's true these products are also processed foods. So they are not first-class foods—those foods most important for developing and maintaining good health. But you are not going to get infections from them. You're not going to be taking cancers into your body from them such as you may from processed meats. Don't make the mistake of lumping all processed foods into the same level of possible risk. Even though you should be trying to get at least 80 percent to 90 percent of your diet from unprocessed, whole, plant-based foods, there is still a huge difference between processed vegetarian meat substitutes and processed meats.

VITAMIN D DEFICIENCY AND CANCER RISK

About twelve years ago, I read in the local newspaper about a Harvard University professor who had carried out an extensive research project in which he collated more than forty different studies that have been conducted studying the relationship between Vitamin D blood levels and the risk of developing cancer. Based on the studies he reviewed, he found that Vitamin D deficiency was associated with about 35 percent of all cancers. Then the newspaper quoted this researcher as saying something so startling to me that I had to read it three times to make sure I wasn't misunderstanding him. He said that having a high Vitamin D level in the blood has more power to *prevent* cancer than cigarette smoking has the power to *cause* cancer!

In other words, if you have a chronically low Vitamin D level, and you choose not to do anything about it, you are at higher risk for developing cancer than is someone who is smoking!

That is an amazing statement. I have been questioned many times when I have repeated it. I've been laughed at by universities professors, but I challenge anyone to disprove that statement, because this is based on the same statistical analysis that is used in all the smoking research. At the very least, don't fail to address the forgotten wellness strategy of maintaining a good Vitamin D blood level. It could literally save your life if you pay attention to it. Of course, I'm not suggesting that if a person optimizes his or her Vitamin D intake, smoking is no longer a major risk factor. My point is that both smoking and low Vitamin D are significant health problems that can be fully eliminated and reversed.

Dr. Cedric Garland of the Morris Cancer Center at the University of California San Diego is a brilliant researcher who has shown that if we assume a general Vitamin D blood level of 25 ng/mL across the board for everyone, increasing that to 40 ng/mL through exposure to sunshine or Vitamin D supplements would decrease cancer risk in general by as much as 30 percent.[18]

Looking at specific cancers, Dr. Garland states that a Vitamin D level of 34 ng/mL, compared to 25, reduces the risk of breast cancer by 30 percent.[19] We know, too, that exercise can reduce breast cancer risk by 30 percent to 50 percent.[20] With a 36 ng/mL Vitamin D blood level, compared to 25, the risk for Type 1 diabetes drops by 25 percent. Some 30,000 individuals in the United States alone are diagnosed each year with Type 1 diabetes.[21] If we could prevent even 25 percent of those cases, wouldn't that be wonderful?

Studies out of Finland, a country that has the highest rate of Type 1 diabetes in the world, followed mothers who gave their children an average of 2,000 units of Vitamin D daily from birth through age ten. The result? These children were 80 percent less likely to get Type 1 diabetes![22]

For hospital patients, just being in a room that has sunlight streaming through the windows can decrease the need for pain medication by 22 percent.[23] Why? Because the sunlight stimulates serotonin production.

The message is that sunlight, this critical wellness strategy that is so unrecognized and underappreciated, is able to potentially prevent, at least in part, any type of autoimmune disease by increasing the Vitamin D blood levels up to at least 30 ng/mL. More than 30 percent of all cancers could be eliminated, as well as many other health problems, by increasing our levels of Vitamin D through prudent exposure to sunlight.

SUNLIGHT AND VITAMIN D

Studies are clear that just ten minutes of sunlight daily, between the hours of 10:00 A.M. and 4:00 P.M. can dramatically increase your level of Vitamin D. This is one reason that many well-meaning health educators, and even clinicians, may discourage Vitamin D supplements. Conventional wisdom is that if you spend just a little time outside in the middle of the day, you will get all the Vitamin D you need. But there is a problem with that view.

As a clinician, I have tested every single one of my patients' Vitamin D levels since reading that newspaper article more than twelve years ago. And I have discovered that even people who are in the sun much of the time often have low Vitamin D blood levels. In early August of last year, a mother brought her 16-year old daughter to my lifestyle medicine clinic. Her symptoms were unexplained depression and fatigue. We did all the labs recommended in Chapter 12. This young lady had been spending lots of time at the beach, was involved in water sports, and participated in summer camps. She had a great tan, yet her Vitamin D level was critically low at 7.5 mg/dL. The minimum reference level is 30. Why would she be low on Vitamin D?

First, people who are spending a lot of time in the sun may be doing so at a time when the angle of the sun's rays is not steep enough to actually electromagnetically transform the cholesterol just under the skin into Vitamin D. That's how your body turns sunlight into Vitamin D. Sunlight electromagnetically transforms cholesterol into Vitamin D. That's a great use for cholesterol!

However, that electromagnetic transformation happens only if you follow something I call "the sun shadow standard." This standard has to do with the height of the sun in the sky. The rule of thumb is that if your shadow is longer than you are tall, the sunlight isn't making any Vitamin D for you. You may be enjoying the warmth. You may be enjoying the psychological benefit of the sunlight. You may be getting all kinds of other benefits. But you are getting zero Vitamin D, because if your shadow is longer than you are tall, the ultraviolet radiation from the sun that is good for you is not intense enough to penetrate the skin and do its job of making Vitamin D.

> There is another reason why so many people who spend a lot of time in the sun still have low Vitamin D blood levels. My good friend, Dr. John Kelly, a family physician who has done extensive research on diabetes, told me one day, "The reason people have such low Vitamin D levels is because they are showering!"

"You're kidding, right?" I responded.

"No," he insisted. "Check it out."

So I began to do some research. And I found that it takes twenty-four to forty-eight hours for the Vitamin D that sunlight has created from cholesterol just under your skin to actually get into your bloodstream and affect your organs. If you take a bubble bath or a shower and soap up really good, guess what happens to your Vitamin D? It washes right down the drain—at least a large part of it does. That's one possible reason so many of us can be Vitamin D deficient, even though we are getting sunlight in the middle of the day.

Sunlight is not a total blessing. Just because ten or fifteen minutes of midday sun is good for us doesn't mean we should go out in the sun for many hours a day all weekend. If we do that, especially when unaccustomed to the sun, and get a sunburn, we're going to be having all kinds of skin damage and other problems. By the way, what do most people do when they go to the beach and hang out there for many hours? Are they eating dark, green leafy vegetables and lots of lycopene-rich tomatoes and carrots and all those antioxidants that protect them against the extra burst of free-radical damage that occurs from extra exposure to sunlight? No. They're having hamburgers, French fries, and a Diet Coke™.

Your body is programmed to try to repair sun damage right away. When you get a little too much sunlight, there is a repair enzyme—DNA polymerase 3—in your body that senses the damage. Too much sunlight can cause gene mutations while the cell is in the process of division. But just before the cell divides, this enzyme clips out that mutation caused by the excessive burst of free-radical damage from too much sunlight. It removes it and replaces it with the right genetic material so that the damage is repaired. But here is the interesting part. *If you have been drinking caffeine, the ability of polymerase 3 to do its repair work can be reduced as much as 50 percent.* In that case, the cell mutation has a much greater chance of not being deleted and replaced. That's yet another reason to take advantage of strategies for good nutrition. If we're eating right, we can actually handle more sunlight without adverse effects. Even so, we need to be prudent not to get too much sun.

HOW MUCH SUNLIGHT IS ENOUGH?

How much exposure to the sun do we need to create adequate levels of Vitamin D in the blood? That depends. The darker your skin pigmentation, the more melanin content you have, and therefore the more sunlight you need in order to make a given amount of Vitamin D.

Someone with darker skin has a natural protection against excessive sunlight, but that also means that he or she needs to be in the sun four, five, six, seven, eight, nine times longer than somebody with fair skin in order to make the same amount of Vitamin D. These individuals can make a lot of Vitamin D, but they need more exposure in the sun to do so, while still using caution and common sense not to get too much sun.

How do you know if you have enough Vitamin D? When I lived in Guam, I used to think that my Vitamin D levels must be fine, because I walked on the beach every afternoon. But when I actually measured my Vitamin D level, I discovered it was 25 ng/mL. I was at high risk for all kinds of problems, simply because I had never realized how important Vitamin D was and how important it was to measure it instead of just guessing.

What did I do? I fixed it. I made sure not only that I was getting prudent sun exposure, but I also began taking Vitamin D supplements so that the next time I checked my Vitamin D, I was between 70 and 100 ng/mL, right where I wanted to be.

You can manage your levels of Vitamin D. But first you have to measure it. You have to know the numbers. The same is true of any number of things. How do you know if your cholesterol is too high? How do you know if your blood pressure is too high or too low? How do you know if your blood sugar is too high or too low? There really is no way to know unless you test. Knowledge is power, and awareness is a call to action.

SEASONAL AFFECTIVE DISORDER (SAD)

Another consequence of not getting enough sunlight is seasonal affective disorder (SAD). An estimated 35 million Americans suffer from this SAD condition that occurs during the winter simply because of a lack of sunlight.[24]

Sunlight is actually a nutrient for the body—not just because it generates Vitamin D, but because the photons in sunlight have a healing quality, psychologically and physiologically. Those with SAD tend to feel sad or irritable and are more likely to become violent. They have decreased physical energy and an increased appetite for carbohydrates. Darkness spurs binge eating. Eating foods that aren't good for you, especially in large amounts, is much more likely if you're not getting enough sunlight.

> Psychologically, dim light lowers inhibitions; it makes us do things that we would not normally do. It lessens our sense of guilt. It leads to compulsive behavior. A standard treatment for depression is to get the depressed person outside into the sunlight.

If for any reason you're unable to get outside in the early morning sunlight, I recommend that you get a light box with a minimum of 10,000 lux bright light and expose yourself to that for fifteen to twenty minutes every morning. That would be a powerful wellness strategy for improving your overall health.

I have a friend who is an executive of an international corporation. He often spends twelve hours in his office and rarely gets outside. Normally dynamic and energetic in a previous job that involved outdoor activity, he wondered if his fatigue, depression, and newly-acquired mental fog were due to a lack of sunlight. So he did a little research and put a high-lux bright light bulb in his office. Within a week, he was restored to his normal happy and energetic self.

CAN I BE GETTING TOO MUCH VITAMIN D?

Between 1988 and 2004, rates of Vitamin D deficiency have climbed steadily. Current estimates are that 70 percent of individuals are deficient in Vitamin D. The data is just too strong to be dismissed by a few recent studies that put together some statistics to minimize the problem or the importance of maintaining a higher Vitamin D blood level. We must pay attention to the big picture.

One of the reasons people are told to stay out of the sunlight is that too much sunlight will cause wrinkles. Yet, the main avoidable health risk behavior that causes wrinkles is smoking. Smoking decreases circulation to the skin and is far and away the greatest cause of premature wrinkles. Exposure to the sun is not a health risk factor in and of itself. The risk arises when we get too much exposure, especially when we aren't eating a diet that helps to create antioxidant barriers against damage from free radicals.

A first-class diet that avoids meat, dairy, and excess fats and sugar while focusing on whole, plant-based foods powerfully protects the skin against wrinkles and skin-related disorders.

Dr. Robert P. Heaney, MD, professor emeritus of medicine at Creighton University in Omaha, Nebraska and one of the world's leading experts in the area of Vitamin D, has said that every baby, child, and adult who is not already paying attention to his or her Vitamin D blood levels, should automatically increase their intake of this important nutrient by at least 2,000 units a day. Such an increase would cause no adverse side effects, but it would dramatically decrease problems from Vitamin D deficiency.

Here is a rough rule of thumb. The average adult male needs about 6,000 units of Vitamin D daily. The average adult female needs about 5,000 units.

There has never been a reported problem or negative side effect associated with those levels. In fact, studies conducted by Dr. Robert Haney have shown that there has never been a documented toxicity to Vitamin D as long as the blood levels were less than 200 ng/mL.[25] So all the concerns you might hear in the media about Vitamin D being toxic are no more valid than talking about water being toxic. While there have been reports of people dying from drinking too much water, there has never been a reported death due to excess Vitamin D,[26] although it was no surprise when one man who was taking 2,600,000 units a day for many months did end up in the emergency room, feeling pretty bad! In that case, an astute ER physician went through the long list of possibilities for someone who was experiencing muscle rigor, tetanus-like reactions, and who was extremely tired. The ER physician tested this man's Vitamin D blood level, and it was 700! You would expect that might happen to someone taking over 2 million units of Vitamin D a day for nearly a year. The physician told him to stop taking this overdose of Vitamin D, and within a few months, the patient was fine.[27]

You're not taking a huge risk by making sure you have sufficient Vitamin D, but you will be giving your body a huge health benefit if you take advantage of what recent research is showing us about the importance of this nutrient.

THE MANY BENEFITS OF VITAMIN D

Some recent research indicates that if your blood levels of Vitamin D are less than 10 ng/mL, and that is true of many people, you have an 80 percent greater risk for cardiovascular disease than if your levels are at least 15 ng/mL.[28] Of course, your Vitamin D level should be at least 30, and ideally 50 to 100 ng/mL.[29] [30]

One of the most effective ways to protect yourself against influenza is to make sure you have sufficient Vitamin D levels.[31] A study was done of African-American post-menopausal women—women who are at very high risk of influenza due to low Vitamin D, partly because their darker skin provides extra protection from the sun. These women, who were given between 800 and 2,000 units of Vitamin D per day for three years, saw their risk of influenza drop by 66 percent just from the therapeutic dose of the vitamin.[32]

Another report published in a peer-reviewed medical journal documented that you can cure or reverse the beginning of a cold or flu by immediately taking 1,000 units of Vitamin D per pound of body weight, per day for three days.[33] For example, if you weigh 100 pounds, take 100,000 units of Vitamin D per day for three days as soon as you feel the symptoms of a cold coming on. You can take half the daily dose in the morning and half in the evening.

VITAMIN D—THE ENABLER OF HEALTH

At an international medical conference, Dr. Robert Heaney, a top researcher and clinician in the area of Vitamin D, asked the audience, "How can the deficiency of a single nutrient produce so many and such diverse health effects?"

Historically if one single thing is said to have benefits for so many health factors, the first thing that comes to mind is: "This must be snake oil. This is quackery." Here is Dr. Haney's answer. He says that Vitamin D is the integral component of the mechanism whereby cells control gene transcription in response to a variety of stimuli. In other words, Vitamin D literally gets in there and changes the way DNA works to optimize your health. It enables your body's optimal response to a broad variety of signals.

It doesn't force anything; it enables. When you have optimal Vitamin D levels in your blood, your body is now able to do what God created the body to do—destroy disease, optimize hormonal balance, and to do all the things that we have been talking about in this chapter.

But if your Vitamin D level is low, your body's ability to fix those things is disabled. Vitamin D doesn't work like a drug that actually forces a certain body mechanism to work. It is an enabler.

Isn't that how we should be working with one another, living our lives in such a way that we enable each other to take advantage of these health and wellness principles? Not forcing anyone to follow them, but enabling people to choose the very best things in life?

Ultimately, Vitamin D unlocks the code, the template that is inside your DNA library, containing the instructions on how to destroy that very virus, that very bacteria, that very cancer, that is within your body. So if you want to enable your body to optimize its fight against disease, one of the most important, but also most neglected, strategies is to take advantage of all the benefits that sunlight and Vitamin D bring to health.

CHAPTER SUMMARY

>> Pure, simple sunlight is like a miracle "drug" that can tremendously increase your health and wellness.

>> Insufficient Vitamin D is a widespread, ongoing health problem across all demographic groups.

>> Lack of sunlight exposure can be the reason you are sad, irritable, sleep poorly, suffer fatigue, and crave carbohydrates.

>> Thirty to sixty minutes of daily exposure to sunlight promotes physical and psychological wellness. During maximum sun intensity between 10 a.m. and 4 p.m., limit your sun exposure to between 15 and 20 minutes.

>> The "Sun Shadow Standard" is a guide for the time of the day that sunlight is intense enough to generate Vitamin D in the skin.

>> Optimal levels of Vitamin D in the blood have more power to prevent cancer than cigarette smoking has the power to cause cancer.

>> More than 30 percent of all cancers could be eliminated by optimizing our levels of Vitamin D.

>> The average child, teenager, and adult is Vitamin D deficient, and more than 80 percent of individuals have inadequate levels of Vitamin D to optimize health.

>> The good news is that no one needs to stay Vitamin D deficient. We can all optimize our level of Vitamin D.

ENDNOTES

1   Kestenbaum, Bryan R., M.D., M.S., "Chronic Kidney Disease Expert Column: Vitamin D Metabolism and Treatment in Chronic Kidney Disease," *Medscape Nephrology*, posted 03/25/2008.

2   In the United States, Vitamin D blood levels are typically expressed in nanograms per milliliter (ng/mL) and occasionally as milligrams per deciliter (mg/dL). In Europe and many other countries, however, they are usually given as nanomoles per liter (nmol/L). To convert ng/mL to nmol/L, multiply the number of ng/mL by 2.5.

3   Jared Reis, Ph.D., Johns Hopkins School of Public Health. Study presented at the 49th conference of the American Medical Association, Palm Harbor, FL, March 10, 2009.

4   Ginde, Adit, et al., "Demographic Differences and Trends of Vitamin D Insufficiency in the U.S. Population, 1988-2004," *Archives of Internal Medicine*, 169.6 (2009): 626-632.

5   Madrid, Eric, *The Vitamin D Prescription: The Healing Power of the Sun & How It Can Save Your Life* (Charleston, SC: BookSurge Publishing, 2009).

6   "Optimizing Patient Cardiovascular Care with the Hunter Heart Profile," a 2014 presentation by Paul Ziajka, M.D., Ph.D., Director of The Florida Lipid Institute; Diplomat of the American Board of Clinical Lipidology; President of the South East Lipid Association.

7   Draeger, A., "Statin Therapy Induces Ultrastructural Damage in Skeletal Muscle in Patients Without Myalgia," *Journal of Pathology*, September, 2006; 210(1): 94-102.

8   Mohaupt, M., "Association Between Statin-Associated Myopathy and Skeletal Muscle Damage," *CMAJ*, July 7, 2009, Vol. 181, Nos. 1-2; doi:10.1503/cmaj.081785.

9   Willich, S., "Increased Morning Incidence of Myocardial Infarction in the ISAM Study: Absence with Prior Beta-Adrenergic Blockade," *Circulation*, 1989; 80: 853–858.

10 Terman, M., "A Controlled Trial of Timed Bright Light and Negative Air Ionization for Treatment of Winter Depression," *Arch Gen Psychiatry*, October 1998; 55(10): 875-882.

11 Fonken, L., et al., "Light at Night Increases Body Mass by Shifting the Time of Food Intake," *Proc Natl Acad Sci*, USA (2010): 107: 18664–18669. doi: 10.1073/pnas.1008734107.

12 Reid, K., et al., "Timing and Intensity of Light Correlates with Body Weight in Adults," *PLoS ONE*, (2014): 9(4): e92251. doi:10.1371/journal.pone.0092251.

13 Figueiro, M., "Light Modulates Leptin and Ghrelin in Sleep-Restricted Adults," *International Journal of Endocrinology*, (2012): 530726. doi: 10.1155/2012/530726.

14 Egan, Kathleen; Sosman, Jeffrey; and Blot, William; "Sunlight and Reduced Risk of Cancer: Is The Real Story Vitamin D?," *Journal of the National Cancer Institute*, 97.3 (2005): 161-163.

15 Levell, N. J., et al., "Melanoma Epidemic: A Midsummer Night's Dream?" *The British Journal of Dermatology*," 161.3 (2009): 630-634.

16 Smedby, K., "Ultraviolet Radiation Exposure and Risk of Malignant Lymphomas," *Journal of the National Cancer Institute*, (2005): 97: 1-11.

17 Egan, K., "Sunlight and Reduced Risk of Cancer: Is the Real Story Vitamin D?" *Journal of the National Cancer Institute,* 97, No. 3 (February 2, 2005): 161-163.

18 Grassroots Health, "Disease Incidence Prevention by Serum 25(OH)D Level," Grassroots Health, March 2010, accessed September 2012, http://grassrootshealth.net/media/download/disease_ incidence_prev_chart_032310.pdf.

19 Garland, Cedric F., et al., "The Role of Vitamin D in Cancer Prevention," *American Journal of Public Health,* 96.2 (2006): 252-261.

20 Howell, A., "Risk Determination and Prevention of Breast Cancer," *Breast Cancer Research,* (2014): 16:446 doi:10.1186/s13058-014-0446-2.

21 National Diabetes Information Clearinghouse, "National Diabetes Statistics, 2011," National Institutes of Health, accessed July 2012, http://diabetes.niddk.nih.gov/dm/ pubs/statistics/index.aspx.

22 Hypponen, Elina, et al., "Intake of Vitamin D and Risk of Type 1 Diabetes: A Birth-Cohort Study," *The Lancet,* 358.9292 (2001): 1500-1503.

23 Walch, Jeffrey M.; Rabin, Bruce S.; Day, Richard; Williams, Jessica N.; Choi, Krissy; and Kang, James D.; "The Effect of Sunlight on Postoperative Analgesic Medication Use: A Prospective Study of Patients Undergoing Spinal Surgery," *Psychosomatic Medicine,* 67, No. 1, (2005): 156–163. doi: 10.1097/01.psy.0000149258.42508.70.

24 Rosenthal, Norman E., *Winter Blues: Seasonal Affective Disorder, What It Is and How to Overcome It* (New York: Guilford Press, 1993), 20–24.

25 Hathcock, J. N., et al., "Risk assessment for Vitamin D," *American Journal of Clinical Nutrition,* (2007): 85:6-18.

26 Bronstein, Alvin C., et al., "2010 Annual Report of the American Association of Poison Control Centers' National Poison Data System (NPDS): 28th Annual Report," *Clinical Toxicology,* 49 (2011): 910-941.

27 Koutkia, Polyxeni; Chen, Tai C.; and Holick, Michael F.; "Vitamin D Intoxication Associated with an Over-the-Counter Supplement," *The New England Journal of Medicine,* 345 (2001): 66-67.

28 Wang, T., "Vitamin D Deficiency and Risk of Cardiovascular Disease," *Circulation,* January 29, 2008: 117(4): 503-511.

29 Grassroots Health, "Disease Incidence Prevention by Serum 25(OH)D Level," March 2010, accessed September 2012, http://grassrootshealth.net/media/download/disease_ incidence_prev_ chart_032310.pdf.

30 Garland, Cedric F., et al., "The Role of Vitamin D in Cancer Prevention," *American Journal of Public Health,* 96.2 (2006): 252-261.

31 Cannell, John, et al., "On the Epidemiology of Influenza," *Virology Journal,* 5 (2008): 29.

32 Aloia J.; Li-Ng, M.; "Re: Epidemic Influenza and Vitamin D," *Epidemiological Infection Journal,* (2007): 135:1095–1096.

33 Cannell, John, et al., "On the Epidemiology of Influenza," *Virology Journal,* 5 (2008): 29.

FIVE

It's a Gut Feeling

OPTIMIZING DIGESTION

AMONG THE MANY FACTORS THAT AFFECT YOUR HEALTH, there is one that is so subtle, so off the radar screen, that many people never think about it. Or if they do, they don't consider it to be a significant factor in the overall picture of their health. I'm referring to digestion.

FIFTEEN YEARS OF PAIN AND WORRY

Let me tell you about a beautiful lady who came to the Lifestyle Medicine Center in Guam where I was practicing some years ago. There was a large picture window in my office, and I saw her getting out of her car with her little daughter. She was tall and slender. She didn't look as if there was anything wrong with her health. I wondered why she was coming to the wellness clinic.

It turned out that she had an appointment with a colleague in the clinic, Dr. Horinouchi. But a couple of weeks later Dr. Horinouchi was on a medical mission trip, screening individuals in the Marshall Islands for diabetes. I was seeing some of his patients while he was out, and this woman was among them. When she showed up in my office two weeks after her initial visit with my colleague, I asked her, "What is Dr. Horinouchi treating you for? Why don't you fill in a little background for me?"

She said, "On my first visit two weeks ago, Dr. Horinouchi asked me to name my favorite food. I thought that was kind of strange. But I told him— deep dish, extra cheese, spinach pizza." (She didn't know that this was a standard "ice breaker" question that Dr. Horinouchi often asked new patients.)

She continued, "Then he asked, 'What is going on with your health? What is the reason you've come to the clinic today?' I explained to him that for the past fifteen years, starting when I was about fourteen, I have been having periodic, debilitating lower pelvic pain."

She went on to tell me that the pain was so bad that her parents were alarmed and took her to the family doctor. He did test after test, trying to figure out what was wrong. Eventually, he referred the girl to a specialist. The specialist did thousands of dollars' worth of tests to make sure he wasn't missing something that was causing all this pain. He couldn't find anything either.

Still, the intermittent pain would come and go every few days. This went on for years. Not only did she have to suffer this debilitating pain that no one was able to diagnose or treat, she also had to deal with the psychological torment of wondering, *What's wrong with me? What could possibly be wrong with me that not even the best doctors around can understand?* And she determined that someday she would find a doctor who would finally be able to discover and explain the problem. She lived in dread that it would turn out to be some rare disease or some cancer, perhaps.

The physical pain and the emotional trauma continued for fifteen years. For all those years, she was convinced that something horrible was wrong with her.

"I explained all this to Dr. Horinouchi," she told me. "He asked me a few more questions, and within five minutes, he said, 'I think I know what is wrong with you.'

"I almost got up and walked out of his office. He hadn't even done any tests on me. He hadn't even looked at my medical history or the records of all the tests that had been done on me in the past. I didn't believe he could possibly know what was wrong with me when all these other experts and specialists had been working with me, on and off, for fifteen years without having a clue about what was causing my pain."

CHANGES IN DIET

But she didn't walk out. Dr. Horinouchi asked her if she would be willing to make a few changes in her diet and come back in two weeks. She reluctantly agreed.

She went on with her story, giving me more insight into her situation. Because of the pain she was experiencing, she had become especially interested in health issues while she was in high school. She read every single book in her high school library that dealt with health. As a result, she became knowledgeable about health issues in a way that most young people her age were not.

When she was 16 years old, she decided to become a vegetarian. Her parents were concerned. Back then, people wondered how vegetarians would be able to get enough protein in their diet to be healthy. "This is a terrible decision," they warned her. "You're going to get worse; you'll become malnourished."

But because of her awareness of health issues and all her reading, she was comfortable with the idea of making the move to a vegetarian diet.

Her parents were encouraged by the fact that she continued to eat dairy products such as milk and cheese, even though she was no longer eating meat. She was getting protein through the dairy products; she was getting enough calories. But her pain persisted.

PAIN FREE!

Now, some fifteen or sixteen years later, she had seen Dr. Horinouchi, and he had asked her to promise to stay away from all dairy and cheese for just ten days. "I'm shocked," she told me. "I can't believe what happened."

"What happened," I asked.

"After one day of no dairy products, after that very first day, I actually slept that whole night without any pain! Dairy products and cheese are my favorite food group; I've eaten them regularly, because I thought that was one of the best things I could eat in conjunction with a vegetarian diet."

Maybe the lack of pain was just a coincidence, she thought. Nagging doubts arose. That would be a normal response for anyone in that situation. *What else was different about that day that could have caused the lack of pain?* she asked herself. She had promised Dr. Horinouchi to eliminate dairy from her diet for ten days to two weeks. And she wanted to keep her promise.

But after a week of no pain, she decided she had to know if dairy products were really making the difference—or if it was something else. You see, an elimination diet is the gold standard of figuring out specific foods or food groups a person may be sensitive to.

> The way these diets work, the way we learn to pinpoint specific problem foods, is to reintroduce a particular food item suspected of causing problems. This is called "re-challenging."

"So, last night," she told me, "I decided I was going to reintroduce my favorite food." She was smiling as she told me this, and I was smiling, because both of us knew where this story was going. She continued, "I made my favorite deep dish, extra cheese spinach pizza. Within an hour of eating it, I was doubled over in pain. And you know, I couldn't decide whether this was a good thing or a bad thing." She was in a lot of pain, but in the back of her mind she was thinking, *Wow! Can this actually be true? Can Dr. Horinouchi have really figured out my problem after just five minutes of assessing my situation and listening to my story?*

Good clinicians often say, "If I just listen to patients long enough, they will tell me exactly what is wrong with them." What do they mean? They mean that by listening and looking at the patterns and putting all that information into the context of their background knowledge, all of a sudden, they start seeing something that has been right in front of the patient for years or decades, but that the patient hasn't picked up.

This lady was just beside herself as she told me her experience. I couldn't take any credit for it. I was only a witness to the aftermath. She went on to tell me that just a month earlier, after six thousand dollars of tests, her specialist had finally told her, "I have no idea what is causing your pain. Why don't you go to the wellness center over there?"

This specialist really had no interest in our approach to health at the wellness center—she just saw it as a final option when all else had failed. But the result was that after fifteen years of pain and emotional distress, this lady no longer had to face the constant physical trauma and the nagging worry that someday some smart doctor would finally figure out the problem and tell her she had some horrible, little-known, incurable disease. She no longer had to face those fears that come in the minutes or hours that you're trying to go to sleep, when you begin thinking of all those things you really don't want to think about.

ON A TIGHTROPE IN HIGH HEELS

What are the issues in your life that keep you awake at night when the fears and worries crowd in and demand to be heard? We all face them. We all have to deal with them. Life is a balancing act. It is hard enough to walk on a tightrope, but doesn't it sometimes feel as if you're having to walk a tightrope in high heels?

The challenge is to make sure that we're taking time for the most important things. But it isn't always easy to determine priorities. We don't always know what the most important things are.

> Good health is important, but not merely as an end in itself. Good health is important because it allows us to live a certain kind of life.

If you sit down and think about it, the most important things in life are relationships—a spiritual relationship with God and a loving, growing relationship with family and those you love the most. That's why good health is so important; it allows you to live a life filled with opportunities to develop and experience those kinds of relationships.

Now, the lady in the story above knew she had a problem, a physical problem. But sometimes the symptoms aren't there, and we aren't aware that we have a problem. That's when important wellness strategies can easily be lost sight of. It's possible to go on year after year, even decade after decade, making the same mistakes and not realizing it. And if we don't recognize a problem, we're not going to address it. We're going to miss dealing with the most important things in life.

When my oldest uncle, Dr. Stephen Youngberg was 80 years old, I drove him to his alumni gathering at Loma Linda University. I said, "Uncle Stephen, how many of your classmates are still alive?"

"Well, last year," he said, "there were thirty of us."

After the meeting, I picked him up. Half-jokingly, I said, "How many of your classmates are left now?"

"We're down to 27," he answered.

"That's a decrease of 10 percent a year," I told him. "You're in a high risk group."

He turned to me and said, "Wes, you never know. You could be walking across the street tomorrow and be hit by a car and killed."

I didn't think much about it that night, but less than ten days later that is exactly what happened to him. But that night, we had the chance for a wonderful talk. "You're 80 years old," I said, "what advice do you have for me?"

He said, "Wes, don't work so hard; spend more time with your family." That's good advice for all of us. Those were his last words to me, and I cherish them.

You know, we get so crazy busy in this fast-paced life we live that we often forget what is most important.

So make sure that whatever you do, whatever strategies you are emphasizing in your wellness program, that first and foremost you are doing it with and for family, because family is the most important thing that we have in this world. Make sure you're doing things for the right reasons.

HIGH-CALORIE MALNUTRITION

Chronic disease or any form of health dysfunction is most often caused by a deficiency of some kind, a missing wellness strategy. Some of the strategies for health and wellness that are most easily overlooked are those that deal with how we access nutrition, how we ensure that we are truly getting the nutrition we think we're getting.

When you look at the typical U.S. food consumption by calories, you begin to get an idea of why there is so much chronic disease, so much health dysfunction, among us. It is because a full 51 percent of the calories consumed by Americans come from refined and processed foods. Processed foods, by their very nature, are nutritionally deficient; they have had the majority of the good things taken out of them. Processed foods promote the modern American paradigm of hyper-caloric malnutrition.

> Americans are getting plenty of calories. In fact, we are getting far too many calories, yet those calories are not satisfying even our minimal nutritional needs. It's no wonder we keep eating more and more on average. Why? Because the body is saying, "I'm still missing something. Keep eating, maybe you'll eat the right thing, and I'll get more nutrients." You see, if we keep eating the same foods that cause that hyper-caloric malnutrition in the first place, we are never going to catch up nutritionally.

Another 42 percent of the average American diet consists of dairy and animal foods. These, too, are processed in their own way. By their very nature, they are not rich in nutrients. Fruits, vegetables, legumes, whole plant-based foods—make up only 7 percent of all the food consumed by Americans. That is a tragedy. It's surprising, given these statistics, that we don't have more chronic disease and more health dysfunction than we do.[1]

80 PERCENT WHOLE, PLANT-BASED FOODS

What should be our goal nutritionally? Instead of getting only 7 percent of our food from whole, plant-based foods, we should be aiming for at least 80 percent! That ought to be the goal. These are "first-class foods." You don't have to limit the amount of these foods in your diet, because they are so loaded with nutrients that every time you eat them, you're significantly improving your genetic potential for health and wellness.

Additionally, refined starches ought not to make up more than 10 percent of your diet, and animal products less than 8 percent. These are some dietary goals you should be trying to reach in order to be healthy. For food lists, sample menus, and details on setting up a first-class diet see the Appendix at the end of this book.

LEGUMES AND COLORFUL VEGETABLES

The big killers in modern society are heart disease and cancer, and nutritional research has shown that eating a lot of vegetables, either raw or cooked, can reduce cancers by 50 percent.[2] That is assuming that these vegetables are actually being broken down in our digestive tracts so that our bodies can assimilate their nutrients. Good digestion is extremely important to good health.

Legumes such as beans, peas, and lentils provide three times more protein and fiber than other starches. In many respects, legumes are the king of all foods, because they are loaded, not only with healthy protein and fiber, but with many of the other vitamins and minerals our bodies need.

But all this nutritional goodness does little or nothing for us if we are not digesting them well. Healthful foods aren't doing us any good at all if we are avoiding them because they don't agree with us.

I am not suggesting that everyone has to eat legumes in order to be healthy. I *am* suggesting, however, that if legumes and other healthy foods don't agree with us, we should be doing our best to understand why and fix the problem of poor digestion.

Six or eight servings daily of non-starchy, low-calorie, colorful vegetables such as raw salads, cruciferous vegetables, greens, and other colorful vegetables, will dramatically increase our ability to reverse disease. Yet, as I pointed out earlier, very few people come close to consuming this amount of vegetables on a daily basis. So we have a lot of growing and improving to do nutritionally.

DIGESTION—A CRITICAL WELLNESS STRATEGY

We eat to supply proper nutrients to every cell in the body so that we can enjoy good health. And that requires a healthy digestive system. The foods that we consume provide the building blocks for every physical process carried out by the body and for every mental function occurring in the brain. That's right, our moods, our emotions, and our mental ability are all strongly affected by the foods we eat and by how well the body is able to extract and utilize the nutrients they contain. That's the role of digestion, and that is why optimizing digestion is such a critical wellness strategy.

One of my medical heroes is Dr. Franz Ingelfinger. Born in 1910, he became a medical doctor and president of the American Association of Gastroenterologists. Dr. Ingelfinger in the 1950s, 60s, and 70s almost single-handedly brought the whole field of gastrointestinal medicine into line with strict scientific protocols. He was an academic, and served from 1967 to 1977 as chief editor of the *New England Journal of Medicine,* which then and now is generally considered to be the foremost medical journal in the world. In that journal, Dr. Ingelfinger reminded his physician colleagues that more than 80 percent of all human illnesses are within the scope of the body's natural healing system. Do you believe that? That was a bold statement for a medical academic to make back fifty years ago. I'm convinced that Dr. Ingelfinger was right; the body has systems in place to heal itself of most of the diseases that befall it.

And I'm convinced that if you follow the wellness strategies in this book and continue to apply the principles that optimize your genetic potential, you will significantly increase that ability your body has to heal itself.

Doctors don't really heal people. I don't heal people. We can facilitate healing, but actual healing is carried out by the body itself. Our bodies were designed and created with this intrinsic ability to heal itself if we will just follow the laws of health. Actually, we need to do more than simply follow the laws of health; we need to embrace them and learn how they work and take advantage of them in every way we can.

Digestion is one of the most important wellness strategies in the body's amazing ability to heal itself. The individuals who come to me, wanting to improve their health, have a variety of medical problems they are experiencing. As I begin working with them, if I have any inkling at all that they may be having digestion difficulties, I stop right there and say, "We need to take care of this before we do anything else."

Often the problem is subtle, and they aren't aware that there is anything amiss with their digestion. "Oh, no," they tell me. "My digestion is fine."

But after another twenty minutes into the initial visit, I am quite clear that their digestion is not fine. And until we can figure out just what the problem is and how to fix it, anything else we might do to improve health and wellness is severely limited

LUCY'S STORY

Lucy had been coming to our wellness program. She was overweight and diabetic. Her blood sugars were out of control; her cholesterol was high; her blood pressure was high. Lucy was a metabolic mess! But she was committed to improving her health. Soon after beginning the program, she started losing weight and her blood sugars came down. She was so excited.

Then about six weeks into the program her blood sugars started coming back up again. She hadn't lost any weight in the previous two weeks, and she was beginning to have some pains.

So I said, "Tell me about your pain? Where are you hurting?"

"I'm not sure," she replied. "I'm concerned I might have kidney cancer. I've already gone to my family doctor. He has done an ultrasound and a CT scan. He's worried about my condition because of my out-of-control diabetes. But he hasn't found any specific problems. In fact, he said I'm actually doing a lot better than I was a few months ago."

I knew she was improved from where she was when she started the program, but she was having these pains. I asked her how she was doing with her diet.

"I'm not eating anything bad for me," she insisted.

But I had a follow up question for her. "Are you eating enough of the healthful foods? The ones that provide the building blocks for healing?" You see, it isn't a question of just avoiding bad things; it's also a question of eating enough good food so that the body will have the necessary building blocks to be able to bring about healing.

As Lucy and I talked, she said, "You know, I haven't been eating beans or non-starchy vegetables for about three weeks." She had not realized it, but whenever she ate those foods, they didn't agree with her so she had been subconsciously avoiding them. By the end of the visit, she realized that she needed to concentrate on fixing her digestion problem.

HOW DIGESTION WORKS

The digestive process is an intricate one. Food goes into the mouth, is chewed and swallowed into the esophagus, from which it flows into the stomach and then into the intestines. How does it all work? How do the different parts of the process fit together to extract the nutrients from our food and turn them into buildings blocks the body can use to grow and fight illness and promote health?

Digestion actually begins in the mouth when we chew our food, mechanically breaking it down. The saliva in our mouths contains an enzyme that begins digesting any starches in the food.

The food then travels down the esophagus and into the stomach. The stomach has three layers of muscles that work like an old fashioned washing machine. Just like those old washing machine churned dirty clothes around and around in soapy water, the stomach's three-layer muscle system, churns the food you've eaten, mixing it with the stomach's gastric juices and initiating the digestion of proteins in the food, preparing it for all the other stages of digestion. The gastric juices are primarily a combination of hydrochloric acid and pepsinogen. Since these two chemicals could damage the stomach and cause an ulcer, the inner lining of the stomach has a mucosal layer of tissue that produces a protective coating of mucus.

After enough time for adequate mixing and the gastric phase of digestion, the stomach muscles begin to move the food mixture, now a thick liquid, into the intestines where more digestive enzymes are released by the pancreas. The intestines are where most of the digestive process takes place ensuring optimal absorption of nutrients. But it's important to note that the more alkaline, intestinal phase of digestion is properly activated only when the food coming from the stomach has been mixed with an optimal amount of hydrochloric acid. So an acidic stomach at meal time will help ensure health by optimizing intestinal absorption of key minerals such as magnesium and potassium that then help maintain an optimal alkalinity in our system. In short, after eating we need an acidic stomach in order to have an alkaline system.

THE IRONY OF ACID INDIGESTION

When this process works the way it is supposed to, the body absorbs nutrients from our food and uses them to keep the body operating properly.

But when the digestive process doesn't function as it should, the symptoms include heartburn, acid indigestion, and Gastroesophageal Disease (GERD). Have you noticed all the prescription and over-the-counter medications for various types of acid indigestion? Obviously, a lot of people are having digestive problems.

It's ironic, because the stomach is supposed to be acidic. It's designed to be an acid producing factory, an enzyme producing factory. It is supposed to be so acidic that optimal stomach pH after eating is between 2 and 3, with 0 and 1 being the most acidic environment possible. Yet at the same time, there is a whole medical industry in place to combat the stomach's acidity.

On one level, of course, it seems to make sense. A person is suffering from symptoms of acid reflux—heartburn, GERD. Or he has an ulcer or gastritis. What's the accepted solution? Take an antacid medication, a proton pump inhibitor, an H2 blocker, or some over-the-counter pill. Yes, these things may relieve symptoms, but what is actually happening to the person's health when he uses these things?

Putting a Band-Aid® on any medical problem places you at greater risk in the long run, because you aren't actually addressing the *cause* of the problem. There are times when it's advisable to take an antacid or a prescription medicine for an ulcer. The problem is that once you begin taking these medicines, you often have a difficult time getting off of them. The studies are very clear. The longer you are on these kinds of medications, the greater the risk that your bone density will be weakened and the likelihood of fractures increases.

In fact, if you have been taking these prescription anti-acid medications during the previous year, you are at a 40 percent greater risk of having a bone fracture this year.[3] If you have been taking them for more than five or seven years, you are at a 400 percent greater risk of suffering a fracture.[4]

Another significant problem with blocking the stomach's acid and interfering with what the stomach was designed to do in the first place, is that now you are unable to destroy bacteria that are present in your food. Bacteria can multiply and start taking over your digestive system. Many individuals, especially the elderly, are coming down with *clostridium difficile*, which is a serious infection causing significant levels of diarrhea that can be fatal. It is a chronic bacterial infection that is often caused by a lack of sufficient acid in the stomach—and a known health risk factor for those taking acid-blocking medications.[5]

Often, for no real reason other than the fact that they are in the hospital, patients are given antacid medication to protect against a potential stress-induced ulcer. Patients are frequently sent home on these medications upon discharge from the hospital. It may seem like a good idea, but in reality it is devastating the health of thousands of individuals, because now it becomes very difficult for them to get off this medication. In the meantime, their digestion is compromised with a decreased ability to absorb key nutrients.

Multiple studies have clearly shown that individuals on antacid medications develop magnesium deficiency.[6] This is such a problem that the FDA has released multiple warnings about long term use of Proton Pump Inhibitor antacid medications.[7]

POOR DIGESTION AND PAIN—A CASE STUDY

Some years ago I was working with the wife of the chairman of the board of a large health insurance company. She was very interested in wellness and had come to the wellness center for help with her prediabetes. She had been encouraging her husband to come to the center also and be checked, but he didn't feel he had time. He considered the things we were doing at the wellness center to be similar to getting a massage—nice, but not terribly important.

But then, at times, he began having a debilitating pain in his mid-section. Just bending over slightly would cause excruciating pain. He went to his family doctor. The doctor, knowing this man was chairman of the board of a major health insurance company, wasted no time ordering all the appropriate tests. But every test came back normal. The doctor ordered additional tests. After several thousands of dollars' worth of tests, he had to tell this man, "Clearly, you have pain in your digestive organs, but we can't find anything that indicates the cause. There is no sign of a tumor, but just to be thorough I am going to refer you to a surgeon."

The surgeon he was sent to happened to be a friend of mine. The surgeon told him, "You know what surgeons do, right? I can cut out your colon, and you won't have any more pain. You also won't have a colon. I am going to refer you to a subspecialist at Loma Linda University."

So this man went to see the subspecialist who told him it would be a crime to have his colon surgically removed. He gave him some medicine, saying, "Take this, and your pain will go away."

He took the medicine, and sure enough, the pain went away. He was good. But two weeks later, he needed a double dose of the medication to get the same relief. After about six months, he was having to take six pills of this medications to deal with the pain in his bowels, but even so he was hurting worse than he had been at the beginning.

Finally, mostly to humor his wife, but also because he was hurting so much, he came to see me at the wellness center. When he walked into my office, he said, "Don't talk to me about diet; my diet is good."

"Alright," I said. I had intended simply to listen to him during that initial visit anyway. I started asking some simple questions. He began telling me his story. Within a few minutes I realized that he had a major digestive issue that could be fixed pretty simply if he would be willing to make a few simple dietary changes. But I bit my tongue and let him talk.

I put him on a few digestive enzymes and a little hydrochloric acid with meals to better acidify his stomach, because his stomach wasn't producing acid properly.

> If your stomach doesn't produce enough acid for whatever reason—and there are many reasons why that might happen—you aren't going to be able to digest your food very well. You are not going to absorb minerals or fat-soluble vitamins very well, and that's a huge problem.

He agreed to go along with my recommendations for a few days. Within two days, he discovered that his wife had been right to urge him to come to the wellness center. His digestion improved, and his pain disappeared. He was very grateful, but of course his wife was even more grateful, because she had been very concerned for his health.

DIET AND EMOTIONS

Is there a connection between what we eat and our emotions? Is it possible that anxiety, even panic attacks, can be related to what we eat or how well we are able to digest our food?

A lady came to see me who had been referred to me by her psychiatrist, because her triglyceride blood levels were over 700. The psychiatrist told her, "I can help you with your panic attacks, but I don't think I can help you with your sky-high triglycerides. You should discuss that issue with someone at the Lifestyle Medicine Clinic."

When she came to see me, she seemed very gregarious. She began telling me about all sorts of things. To me, she didn't fit the profile of someone who was overly anxious. I started asking a few questions, "When do these panic attacks occur?"

"Oh, they can occur anytime."

Now, I know that often we are not aware of what is happening in our own bodies. So I asked her the same question three or four different ways.

Finally, she paused and said, "You know, these panic attacks usually happen about an hour after dinner."

That was a big clue that some subtle digestive issue was taking place. When we eventually determined exactly what was causing her problems, we discovered that her stomach lining was not producing hydrochloric acid the way it is supposed to. She wasn't breaking down foods properly in her stomach. Instead, without the optimal amount of digestive juices and hydrochloric acid, the carbohydrates in her food quickly began to ferment in her stomach. This produced lactic acid[8] and pyruvic acids in a gas form that were creating bloating and pressure underneath her rib cage. This buildup of lactic acid gas in the digestive system can then easily perfuse into the blood stream, cross the blood/brain barrier, and stimulate the amygdala. In sensitive individuals this causes a chemically induced panic attack.[9] [10] That was what was happening with this lady. By properly addressing her digestion, this patient had a dramatic improvement in the frequency and intensity of her panic attacks.

I'm not suggesting that panic attacks are primarily caused by poor digestion. But I believe that in many cases it is a contributing factor.

I've seen many people experience significant improvement in their emotional outlook when they become aware of how good digestion relates to our moods, our emotions, and the potential for anxiety attacks.

POOR DIGESTION AND THE BODY'S NEED FOR MINERALS

One symptom of poor digestion is low blood minerals. Minerals are important to many body functions, and not having enough minerals can cause a variety of health problems. For this reason, doctors may recommend testing levels of minerals free flowing in the blood serum. Optimally, we want to know how well minerals have been assimilated into the tissues where they are used for many physiological functions. To test the level of minerals inside the cells, clinicians can order a Red Blood Cell (RBC) Mineral Profile, thus providing specific nutritional guidance for that patient.

Your immune system depends on having a sufficient supply of certain minerals in order to operate as efficiently as possible. Poor digestion, due to not having enough acid in the stomach, means your body can't utilize the magnesium, chromium, or selenium in your food very well. These are minerals your circulatory and immune systems need to function effectively.

Your risk of having a heart attack dramatically increases if you are not able to absorb magnesium as you should.[11] The vast majority of Americans are deficient in magnesium.[12] That is not a theory; it is a fact that has been proven over and over by government studies.

One reason is that we aren't eating enough whole, plant-based foods that are rich in magnesium. But we are also magnesium deficient because of poor digestion which makes it difficult for our bodies to assimilate magnesium and other nutrients as they should.

Many people try to make sure they are getting enough vitamins and minerals by taking supplements. When done with the proper testing and guidance, this is not only rational but also prudent. However, when they develop stomach discomfort or other negative symptoms, they may think that vitamin and mineral supplements aren't good for them. It's more likely, however, that the real problem is not having enough acid in their stomach to properly assimilate the vitamins, and especially the minerals, in that pill. Their discomfort is actually a sign that they are in real need of these nutrients. But the permanent solution is to fix the digestion problems so that their body can also more effectively get its needed vitamins and minerals from the food they eat.

For instance, I often see patients with clear signs and symptoms of chromium deficiency. They may have tendencies to hypoglycemia—low blood sugars, prediabetes, diabetes, and other conditions associated with insulin resistance. But if they experience nausea or stomach pain when supplementing chromium, I quickly suspect hypochlorhydria—a condition in which the stomach is currently not producing adequate amounts of hydrochloric acid (HCL).

There are many more examples that demonstrate our great need for optimal amounts of minerals. Few of us are aware that the mineral, magnesium, can be a powerful nutritional strategy in preventing and treating a long list of conditions, including headaches, constipation, diabetes, anxiety, and depression. With proper guidance, magnesium citrate or Kreb's magnesium can be taken at bedtime and more often throughout the day as needed. Low magnesium levels are also a primary cause of cholesterol-forming plaque. Harvard studies have shown that if you have an optimal blood level of magnesium, you won't have the amount of artery plaque development typically associated with a higher cholesterol.[13] But as soon as magnesium levels fall, plaque begins to form and create atheromas in the arteries.[14] So optimizing digestion can be a critical step in preventing heart disease.

Ulcers and liver problems are caused by poor digestion. Digestion is a factor even in bone spurs! Bringing magnesium levels up to normal is a key step in resolving bone spurs or preventing them from becoming worse. Poor digestion is definitely a factor in diabetes. Improving digestion will typically lower blood sugars even if there is no change in caloric intake or exercise.

MEALTIME—WHEN AND HOW OFTEN?

When are the best times to eat and how many meals should we eat each day in order to optimize health and wellness? These are major questions in terms of digestion. The number of meals you eat in a day has a powerful influence on your body's ability to digest that food. Obviously, quality is critical. Eating healthful, first-class foods with each meal is much more important than when or how often you eat. But assuming a healthful diet, how many meals a day should the average person eat?

> In general, you should eat two or three meals a day with at least four or five hours between meals. This is especially true if you're sedentary most of the day or if you're trying to lose weight, lower your triglyceride fats, or lower your blood pressure or blood sugars.

Of course, there are always exceptions to any rule. If you are diabetic and you are taking insulin or other diabetes medications, you don't want to let your blood sugars get too low. That is far worse than letting them get high. You want to protect against low blood sugars. If you tend to be hypoglycemic, you don't want to eat only two meals a day. If you are trying to rebuild your adrenals and support stabilization of blood sugars, you will probably want to eat three meals a day, but make sure those meals are well balanced. One of the biggest challenges to good digestion is that meals often aren't well balanced with enough healthy proteins, healthy fats, and healthy high fiber carbohydrates. If you need help on how to do this, see the appendix at the end of this book.

The most important time to eat is breakfast. If you don't feel like eating breakfast, that suggests that you have a digestive problem. It's possible that food from the night before is still "sitting there" in your stomach or that your stomach has not yet recovered from digesting that late evening meal or bedtime snack. Not wanting to eat breakfast is something you need to fix right away. For some people, that will mean not eating an evening meal. Or it may mean eating a lighter, earlier dinner, preferably before 7:00 P.M. There should be at least three hours, preferably four, between dinnertime and bedtime. It takes that long to ensure that you aren't going to bed with your stomach still processing food. If your stomach is still working when you go to bed, you aren't going to sleep well, and you aren't going to get that restorative sleep that is so critical to health and healing.

> To begin eating breakfast, some people will need to go for a week or two without an evening meal. It isn't easy, but you won't starve! You will feel a lot better if you start eating a regular breakfast and a good lunch—and if necessary, a lighter, earlier evening meal.

OPTIMIZING DIGESTION

Hydration is critical to good digestion. But drinking with meals isn't the best way to keep your body hydrated. In fact, habitually drinking more than a few ounces of liquids with your meal—especially lots of cold, icy, liquids— could lead to unhealthful levels of fermentation byproducts in the stomach. You should drink water at least a half hour before you eat your meal. Then your stomach will be better prepared to digest your food properly and produce an optimal concentration of digestive enzymes and hydrochloric acid that will break down and support the assimilation of the nutrients in your food.

Don't wash down your meal with water—and certainly not with soda!

My experience suggests that the best approach is to drink a tall glass of water the first thing in the morning. Then drink more water about an hour and a half after breakfast. Drink again a half hour before your next meal and repeat this pattern throughout the day. This will ensure that you stay hydrated and also that you will be optimizing your digestion and circulation. Without enough water in your system, you are going to be dehydrated and your circulation will be impaired. Risk of a stroke or heart attack increases if you don't get enough water throughout the day.

Stroke patients and those with TIAs ("transient ischemic attacks" or mini-strokes) are typically diagnosed by their emergency room doctor as having high plasma osmolality levels and volume depletion.[15] That's a fancy way of saying, "You're dehydrated!" Drinking six glasses of water daily, or more, is a major simple step to being healthy.

If you don't like water, learn to like it! There really is no healthful substitute for water. You can add a twist of lemon or lime to it if you wish, but for good digestion and good health, you must learn to enjoy water. Don't think that coffee can take the place of water and keep you hydrated. Coffee is actually a diuretic and promotes dehydration. It also increases your risk of coronary heart disease.[16] Since caffeine increases the amount of cortisol released, both at rest and when under stress,[17] it is easy to see how morning use of coffee or other forms of caffeine will increase the risk of morning heart attacks. Morning is the time of day we are most dehydrated and the time our stress hormone, cortisol, is at a high point.

For some people, optimizing digestion may mean eliminating dairy products from their diet. Others might be sensitive to wheat, eggs, or corn. If you're having symptoms, quit eating the suspected food products for three weeks and then re-challenge by adding specific items back into the diet and see what items are causing problems for you.

Digestion can be improved for some by taking a little warm liquid just before eating a meal. A small amount of warm soup or some warm herbal tea will prepare your digestive track for better digestion. Some people find that limiting the number of different foods eaten in a single meal is helpful to digestion. Avoid irritating foods. We're all different in our reactions to specific foods, so pay attention to your body and avoid foods that you know are irritating to you.

No discussion of digestion would be complete without looking at the role of charcoal in the digestive process. Charcoal, used right, is a medical marvel. It is a way to clean up toxins in your system. Charcoal is like a black hole; it sucks up nearly anything that has the potential to be toxic to your body. You can take a teaspoon to a tablespoon of activated charcoal mixed into four to six ounces of cold water, but be sure to do so at least two hours *before* or at least three hours *after* any medications, because charcoal will bind to almost any medicine you take. There is nothing better than charcoal to clear up an intestinal infection, a viral or bacterial stomach flu, or a toxin that has gotten into your system.

For a full and very practical clinical discussion on optimizing digestion, read chapter 14 of my book, *Goodbye Diabetes*. Whether you are trying to reverse a chronic disease or simply optimize your genetic potential, fixing digestion is of utmost importance.

A CALL TO ACTION

Did you notice that in each of the case studies presented in this chapter, the person suffering from digestion problems didn't believe that their symptoms had anything at all to do with digestion? Most of these individuals were quite knowledgeable about health and medical issues—more so in many instances than the average person. Yet they dismissed digestion as a cause of their health problems. It's easy to overlook the role that digestion plays in health and wellness. But never think that you can't dramatically improve your health by paying attention to your digestion!

Here is the challenge. Will you go on doing things as you always have? Or will you invest the time and effort necessary to become aware of how you can feel better, live more healthfully, and enjoy life more?

Remember, more than 80 percent of all human illness is within the reach of the body's natural healing system. That statement is a call to action. Will you optimize your digestion and give your body the nutrients it needs to heal itself? Will you follow a program that is based on what is best for you and your family?

CHAPTER SUMMARY

>> The food we consume provides the building blocks for every physical and mental function of our bodies. That's why optimizing digestion is such a critical wellness strategy.

>> More than 80 percent of human illness can be healed naturally by the body, but only if the proper healing strategies are followed.

>> Poor digestion can affect your emotions.

>> Most people should eat two or three meals a day with four or five hours between meals.

>> Breakfast is the most important meal of the day.

>> Drinking at least six glasses of water daily is a major step toward being healthy. But drinking with meals is not the best way to stay hydrated.

>> Long term use of acid-blocking medications can increase the risk of bone fractures more than 400 percent.

>> Minerals, especially magnesium, deficiency is very common and powerfully promotes our risk for developing many health problems, including depression, anxiety, diabetes, headaches, heart disease, muscle cramps, and constipation.

>> Good health is important, but not merely as an end in itself. It is important because it allows us to live a life filled with loving, growing relationships with God, family, and friends.

>> Refined and processed foods account for more than half of the calories consumed by Americans; dairy and animal foods make up more than 40 percent; and only 7 percent comes from whole, plant-based foods—fruits, vegetables, and legumes.

>> Ideally, at least 80 percent of your diet should be whole, plant-based foods. Refined starches should not make up more than 10 percent of your diet, and animal products less than 8 percent.

>> Eating lots of vegetables, either raw or cooked, can reduce cancers by 50 percent.

ENDNOTES

1　Joel Fuhrman, *Eat to Live: The Revolutionary Formula for Fast and Sustained Weight Loss,* (Boston: Little, Brown, 2003), 187.

2　Key, T., "Fruit and Vegetables and Cancer Risk," *British Journal of Cancer,* (2011): 104, 6–11.

3　Yang, Y., "Long-Term Proton Pump Inhibitor Therapy and Risk of Hip Fracture," *Journal of the American Medical Association,* (2006): 296 (24): 2947-2953.

4　Richards, J., "Proton Pump Inhibitors: Balancing the Benefits and Potential Fracture Risks," *Canadian Medical Association Journal,* August 12, 2008, vol. 179, no. 4, doi: 10.1503/cmaj.080873.

5　Smith, A., "Proton Pump Inhibitors and Clostridium Difficile Infection," *Clinical Correlations, The NYU Langone Online Journal of Medicine,* March 20, 2014.

6　Danziger, J., "Proton Pump Inhibitor Use Is Associated with Low Serum Magnesium Concentrations," *Kidney International,* April, 2013; 83(4):692-699. doi: 10.1038/ki.2012.452. Epub 2013 Jan 16.

7　http://www.fda.gov/Drugs/DrugSafety/ucm245011.htm.

8　Cranwell, P. D., "Gastric Secretion and Fermentation in the Suckling Pig," *British Journal of Nutrition,* July, 1976; 36(1):71-86.

9　Ziemann, A. E., "The Amygdala Is a Chemosensor That Detects Carbon Dioxide and Acidosis to Elicit Fear Behavior," *Cell,* November 25, 2009; 139(5):1012-1021. doi: 10.1016/j.cell.2009.10.029.

10　Maddock, B., "Panic Attacks as a Problem of pH," *Scientific American,* May 18, 2010.

11　Purvis, J., "Magnesium Disorders and Cardiovascular Diseases," *Clinical Cardiology,* August 15, 1992; (8):556-568.

12　Ervin, R., "Dietary Intake of Selected Minerals for the United States Population: 1999-2000," *Advance Data,* April 27, 2004; (341):1-5.

13　Del Gobbo, L., "Circulating and Dietary Magnesium and Risk of Cardiovascular Disease: A Systematic Review and Meta-Analysis of Prospective Studies," *American Journal of Clinical Nutrition,* July, 2013; 98(1): 160–173.

14　King J, "Inadequate Dietary Magnesium Intake Increases Atherosclerotic Plaque Development in Rabbits," *Nutrition Research,* May 29, 2009; (5):343-349.

15　Rodriguez, G., "The Hydration Influence on the Risk of Stroke (THIRST) Study," *Neurocritical Care,* (2009): 10(2):187-194. doi: 10.1007/s12028-008-9169-5. Epub 2008 Dec 3.

16　Cornelis, M., "Coffee, Caffeine, and Coronary Heart Disease," *Current Opinion in Clinical Nutrition and Metabolic Care,* November, 2007; 10(6):745-751.

17　William, L., "Caffeine Stimulation of Cortisol Secretion Across the Waking Hours in Relation to Caffeine Intake Levels," *Psychosomatic Medicine,* (2005): 67(5): 734–739.

Stressed Out

STRESS, EMOTIONS AND ADRENAL FATIGUE

OUR EMOTIONS HAVE THE POTENTIAL TO POWERFULLY influence aspects of our health. What happens in the mind affects the body. And the reverse is true, as well. What happens in the body affects the mind. Here is how one author expresses that idea:

> "The relationship that exists between the mind and the body is very intimate. When one is affected, the other sympathizes. The condition of the mind affects the health to a far greater degree than many realize. Many of the diseases from which men suffer are the result of a mental depression. Grief, anxiety, discontent, remorse, guilt, distrust, all tend to break down the life forces and invite decay and death.
>
> "Disease is sometimes produced and is often greatly aggravated by the imagination. Many lifelong invalids might be well if they only thought so."[1]

THE MIND-BODY CONNECTION

I read that book many years ago, and it changed my understanding of many things. Notice that this statement doesn't say that disease is *always* caused by what we're thinking—our fears, our negative emotions—or that *all* disease originates in the mind. It says that disease is *sometimes* caused by the mind and that negative emotions and thoughts can greatly aggravate disease. In other words, our emotions have the potential to powerfully influence aspects of our health. What happens in the mind affects the body, and what happens in the body affects our mind.

Now, you may be thinking, *That doesn't sound very scientific. That seems a little mystical.*

But the link between our mental attitude and our health is real. And that's good news, not bad news. Henry Ford said, "Whether you think you can or you think you can't, you're right."

You see, if you think you can't, you're not going to put any effort into it; you're not going to try. But if you think you can, you're going to give it your best and stick with it until you've done it. It really is true, as Thomas Edison remarked, "Genius is 1 percent inspiration and 99 percent perspiration." Some people imagine that every slight exposure is going to cause illness, and sure enough, they are often sick. Others assume they are going to be well, and they usually are. The mind has a powerful effect on the body.

The statement from *Ministry of Healing* goes on to declare: "In the treatment of the sick, the effect of mental influence should not be overlooked. Rightly used, this influence affords one of the most effective agencies for combating disease."[2]

I believe that the mind-body connection is one of the foundation stones of health and wellness. It's also a basic concept to nutritional medicine. There is a powerful relationship between our thoughts and what we end up eating. Likewise, what we eat affects our thinking.

YOU ARE WHAT YOU THINK

The proceedings for the National Academy of Sciences, one of the most prestigious scientific organizations in the world, published an amazing study by Dr. Richard Davidson, head of the Laboratory for Affective Neural Science at the University of Wisconsin. The study looked at attitudes of resentment versus attitudes of joy and showed that a person's physical condition reflects his or her thoughts.[3]

Dr. Davidson studied middle-aged women who had come in to get their annual flu shots. Seven minutes before receiving the shot, the women were divided into two random groups. One group was told to think about some wonderful experience in their past, something that gave them a sense of joy and pleasure. They were told to write down a few thoughts about that experience. The second group was asked to do the same—except that they were told to focus on and write about a past experience that had caused them bitterness and resentment. Only seven minutes. Then both groups received their flu shots.

Six months later, both groups of women returned for a blood test that examined how well their flu shot had been able to stimulate the production of antibodies against the expected strain of influenza for that year.

What Dr. Davidson discovered was that, compared to the results for the women who had focused on a positive, pleasurable experience, the women who had focused on negative, bitter emotional experiences—for only seven minutes—had significantly fewer antibodies in their immune system to combat the flu virus.

That's the power of the mind! If we don't control our thoughts, our thoughts will control us.

ACTIVE AND PASSIVE STRESS

In 2008, Dr. Dean Ornish once again amazed the medical community by publishing a study that has challenged the perception of what is possible in medicine. Fifteen years or so earlier, he had shown that heart disease was reversible. The evidence had been there for decades. Numerous animal studies had shown that heart disease could be reversed, but the medical community had not accepted the idea until Dr. Ornish did a study on humans proving it was possible. Now, in the 2008 study, Dr. Ornish was demonstrating that even in cancer patients, the body can modify how the genes express themselves.[4]

In this study involving thirty men, Dr. Ornish applied the very same strategies he had used to show that heart disease could be reversed and applied them to men who had been diagnosed with early prostate cancer. The patients were given a choice: surgery or "watchful waiting"—basically monitoring the disease and waiting to see what happened. Watchful waiting is the more popular option today for early prostate cancer. For many, that may be a better option.

> Watchful waiting is different than merely waiting. Just sitting around waiting to see what happens creates passive stress. It depresses the immune system and makes it more likely the cancer will grow. In fact, passive stress makes it more likely *any* disease will grow worse. Passive stress is really bad for you. Active stress, on the other hand, is actually good for you.

What is active stress? Active stress is when you say, "I understand I have a problem. I'm going to do what I can about it. I'm going to learn more about my health. I'm going to do broader health testing. I'm going to look at my blood work and find where the gaps are." That kind of attitude is critical, especially for someone with cancer. Individuals with cancer often accept the falsehood that all they can do is get treatment. I've talked to cancer support groups many times. These cancer patients often say, "I'm doing all I can. I'm getting this treatment; I'm getting that treatment."

"No!" I tell them. "You're not doing everything you can. There are all kinds of things you could be doing right now. Are you exercising?"

"No. I have cancer."

"That's all the more reason to exercise. You don't have to exercise vigorously. But make exercise part of your daily schedule. How are you doing with your diet?"

"It's too late to change my diet. I already have cancer."

"So, you've just given up?"

You see, when you are diagnosed with cancer or you develop some other medical problem—that's the time you should feel the most motivated and want to make appropriate changes.

That's when you want to do everything reasonable and prudent that you can to help your body combat this disease. That is active stress.

It's good for you. It dramatically enhances your immune system.

WELLNESS STRATEGIES FOR REVERSING DISEASE

In his study of these thirty early prostate cancer patients, Dr. Ornish presented four main wellness strategies they were to follow as they "watchfully waited" the course of the disease. First, he put them on a 100 percent plant-based diet. This diet is known to help reverse heart disease; maybe it would help with prostate cancer.

Second, they were to spend an average of thirty minutes a day in moderate exercise. He didn't expect them to run a marathon. He just wanted them to get outside and do something active.

Third, he taught them stress management techniques. He showed them how to carve out certain times during the day when they could stop the busyness, the rat race, the frantic pace of modern life and focus on relaxing and being calm.

Finally, he involved them in a weekly support group where they could talk about the disease and how they were feeling, mentally and physically. A support group may sound touchy-feely and not very effective in dealing with disease, but it has been shown to be a very important strategy. A study conducted about twenty years ago at the University of California San Francisco Medical Center followed two groups of women who had been diagnosed with terminal breast cancer. Both received the same medical treatment and care. One group met once a week to talk about the disease and how they were feeling and coping. That group lived, on average, about twice as long as the women who weren't involved in a support group.[5]

Dr. Ornish's study involved these four strategies in relation to early prostate cancer—diet, exercise, stress management, and a support group.

The study was designed to look at how genes can change their expression in men undergoing intensive nutrition and lifestyle intervention. What happened?

In three months, forty-eight disease-preventing genes that had been turned off at the beginning of the study were now all turned back on. At the start of the study, biopsies of the prostate gland in these thirty men had determined that these genes were turned off; their disease-preventing characteristics were inactive. But now, only three months later, these genes were back on, like a dimmer switch growing brighter and brighter. It's not just a matter of being on or off; it's a continuum. It's a matter of which direction we're stimulating these genes in their expression.

> Genes actually can control our health in beneficial ways but only if the good genes are turned on and the bad genes are turned off.

Dr. Ornish went on to show that not only had the expression of these forty-eight disease-*preventing* genes been reversed, but so had the expression of 453 genes which are known to *promote* such diseases as breast cancer and prostate cancer. These 453 disease-causing genes had all been turned on at the beginning of the study; three months later they were all turned toward the off position. There was an amazing reversal of both good genes and bad genes in just three months.

The question for us is this: In which direction are our genes being stimulated by our current health and wellness strategies? I've been given the privilege to start working on a research project in which we will be looking at positively reversing gene expression in 120 diabetic individuals. We want to test not just before and after three months, but also after one month, six months, and one year. Why? Because I firmly believe it doesn't take three months to turn on your good genes and turn off your bad genes. I believe it happens within days and weeks, but not switching on or off suddenly—more like the continuum of a dimmer switch. I believe that as long as we maintain optimal wellness strategies, our "bad" genes will stay turned off, and our "good" genes will stay turned on.

STRESS MANAGEMENT AND BLOOD SUGARS

Some time ago I attended a medical conference organized around the theme of preventing diabetes throughout the lifespan. There was a pharmacist at the convention—a great speaker who had had Type 1 diabetes his whole life and was giving himself insulin three times a day. He consistently checked his blood sugar seven times a day—before and two hours after the start of each meal and again at bedtime. Now, when you check some aspect of your body physiology on a regular basis for weeks, months, and years, it gives you a whole new sense of control over your health. It's essentially a form of biofeedback. We know that through biofeedback, by focusing on some aspect of your physiology, you can actually change that physiology.

By checking his blood sugar before and after meals over a long period of time, this pharmacist knew what foods he could handle and what foods increased his blood sugar. But eventually, something unexpected happened. We call it the serendipitous effect of doing the right thing.

> When you start paying attention to your health, you often start seeing new patterns that you would never have seen otherwise.

The pharmacist was keeping a diary of what he was eating. He was writing down whether or not he had exercised that day, because moderate exercise right after eating can lower blood sugar by one to three points for every minute you spend exercising. So he was paying attention to what he was doing to see what worked.

And then he started seeing a new pattern. It was the basis of his lecture at the medical conference. "On the days that I argued with my wife," he told us, "my blood sugars would always be about fifty points higher than they otherwise would have been." He spoke about the impact of stress on diabetes and other functions of our bodies. He went on to explain that when he argued with his teenage daughter, his blood sugars went up *ninety* points higher than normal! This demonstrates how our perception of stress and our level of control in given situations—as well as the amount of frustration we are experiencing—can powerfully influence many of our body systems without our realizing it.

You don't have to be diabetic for stress to affect your blood sugars. I guarantee that stress affects your blood sugars whether or not you're diabetic or prediabetic.

That's one reason, by the way, that stress can cause weight loss, because it creates an environment for some people in which they don't feel like eating. But for other people, stress causes their weight to shoot up. Why? How can stress stimulate food cravings? One way is that stress stimulates the release of cortisol which, in turn, stimulates the liver to dump sugar into the bloodstream.

When this happens, the pancreas starts producing large amounts of insulin to try to counteract the higher blood sugar. The extra insulin stimulates the cells to take in more sugar. This extra sugar is then converted into fat. Ironically, fatter cells increase insulin resistance, which then makes you more sensitive to the bad effects of too much stress and cortisol. It becomes a vicious cycle. So if you're trying to lose weight or lower blood sugars, blood pressure, or blood fats, you want to learn how to manage stress in your life. Stress management is all about self-control—about how well you manage the stressors in your life and the frustrations when things don't go as planned.

UNDERESTIMATING THE STRESS IN OUR LIFE

A woman was referred to me by her family doctor, because her blood sugars were 350—extremely high. As I began talking to her, I could see the tension in her face, in her shoulders. It was obvious to me that she was under a tremendous amount of stress. So I said, "Tell me about your life. What's going on?"

She explained that there were financial difficulties at home. Now, when you have financial problems, what happens between husbands and wives? A lot of arguments and misunderstandings.

Their finances had grown worse, she said, and they lost their home. She and her husband couldn't live together anymore, because they couldn't handle the emotional stress. They had gotten a divorce. Everything about her life had slipped away except her job.

As we were discussing her high blood sugar levels, she said, "My family doctor prescribed an antidepressant for me, but I don't know if I should take it. What do you think?"

I said, "If your family doctor prescribed it for you, you should talk to him. Maybe you need it for a little while until we can properly address the underlying factors causing your depression."

A week later, she came back to see me, because I was having her check her blood sugars frequently. She said, "It's amazing. As soon as I started taking the antidepressant my blood sugars dropped fifty points on average."

Her blood sugars needed to come down a lot more than just fifty points. But what this showed was that as soon as a person is feeling less stressed, for whatever reason, the body begins to turn down the "alarm reaction" to a lower level, and then the blood sugars, blood pressure, triglycerides, weight— all these things start improving.

At work one day, a coworker pulled this woman aside and said, "You've got to get a grip on yourself or you're going to lose your job."

"What are you talking about?" she wanted to know. "I can't lose my job. It's the only thing I have left."

"You're coming across so hostile to everybody in this hospital that you're going to lose your job if you don't change," her coworker confided.

Telling me about this, the woman said, "I had no idea I was wearing all the stress in my life on my shirt sleeve."

You see, when we're under stress, we often don't realize it or we don't realize how severe it is. During stress or any kind of acute emotional difficulty, lower-brain functions tend to shut down higher-brain functions.

The frontal lobe of the brain is where reasoning and establishing priorities and decision-making occurs. This is the function of the "higher" brain. Lower-brain functions are those that aren't concerned with long-term consequences. They are the immediate reactions to external stimuli—"That looks really tasty, so I want it now!" or "I want to do what I feel like doing!" This phenomenon of seeking "instant gratification" is well understood in the field of psychology.

The lower brain doesn't consider how we will feel about our choices tomorrow. It's motivated only by what looks, feels, and tastes good right now! When we're under a lot of stress, our frontal lobe isn't working well, and we need to try to get it back. We need to be trying to understand how we can place the higher brain in charge more of the time and suppress the anxiety and cravings of the lower brain. I often remind myself to do today what tomorrow I'll wish I had done today! In other words, tomorrow, when I look back at what I did today, will I feel guilty or proud of the decisions I made?

Is there anything we can do to manage stress and get it under control?

RESTORING THE INNER SELF

When I talk about stress, I'm talking about something I experience personally. Like some many people these days, I find myself spread too thin at times, stretched out between patients, research, seminars, travel, and challenges of all kinds. Sometimes it all gets to be too much. I need to guard against that, and so do you.

One specific week was like that. I got up at 4:30 on Friday morning to fly from San Diego to Seattle, where I caught a connecting flight to Anchorage. From there I drove to Palmer, Alaska, to hold a three-part health seminar over the weekend. It was a wonderful experience, but at the end of the series of talks, my battery was running low!

On Saturday night, the local coordinator for the series asked if I would like to go flying over a glacier the next morning. All of a sudden, I felt my vital reserves coming back.

Sunday morning, we climbed into a Lake Amphibian and flew for half an hour to land on a frozen lake right next to the glaciers. We spent the next two hours walking around the glaciers, being in nature, and seeing the glory of God in these magnificent ice fields. We found a large ice cave to explore. It was the most amazing cathartic release of stress that I've experienced in a long time. Spending time in the outdoors, enjoying the beauties of nature, is one of the best ways we can relax the stress built up from living in the modern, fast-paced world of today.

Instead of taking advantage of these natural gifts for managing stress, it seems we are all too often intent on finding some shortcut, some short-term solution to our stressful lives. Unfortunately, these shortcuts often make us more stressed in the long run. We need to pay attention to the forms of stress management that not only work now but that continue to enhance vitality and health over time.

As I was walking through that blue ice cave in Alaska, it reminded me of the description we're given by Ezekiel of God's throne, appearing like a translucent sapphire stone.[6] The ice cave in that glacier was like translucent sapphire everywhere I looked—above, below, and all around me. It seemed as if I could have been right there at the base of the throne of God where the River of Life flows out to water the Tree of Life!

That experience made me realize that the way most of us live our lives is so artificial. It's removed from real nature, real healing, real restoration. Just two hours out in nature restored me. I was amazed.

So we need to bring balance back into our lives, to carve out time for restoring our inner self. That's why I personally set aside every Saturday, the last day of the week, as a time for mental, physical, and spiritual rejuvenation. And I don't let anything else crowd out that commitment. I'm still learning how to minimize stress during the rest of the week, but at least I have that weekly respite, that opportunity for personal restoration.

It's a time to build up meaningful relationships with family, help those in need, spend time in nature, and celebrate a time set aside to grow spiritually.

DIET AND BEHAVIORAL CHANGE

Some years ago I was listening to Dr. Dean Ornish answer questions after a lecture. People were asking, "How can we know what part of your treatment was responsible for the results? You were doing all these different things. How do we know nutrition was really that important?"

"First of all," he replied, "everything we did was based on science. We looked at all the studies. What is beneficial from a lifestyle perspective to improve health? And if it was a beneficial factor, we included it. Exercise, nutrition, lifestyle variables, supplements—if it is a prudent strategy, why not do it? If there's good evidence with little risk, do it. Stop saying, 'We need more research to figure this out.' Every researcher says that. Don't believe it. We researchers just want to keep doing research, it's what we do. The reality is that we have a lot of data. We need to start taking advantage of that data now and not wait another twenty years for more research."

Dr. Ornish believes that learning to manage stress is by far one of the most important strategies, if not the most important strategy for wellness. And I agree with him.

There was a study published in the British *Journal of Psychiatry* conducted by Drs. Gash, Hammond, Hansen, and Crowder.[7] They studied a sample of young men in prison. These were violent offenders who were in prison because they were so impulsive they couldn't control their anger. They divided these young men into two groups in a double-blind study. In addition to the standard prison diet, one group got mineral supplements and a capsule of fish oil. The other group received a placebo.

When I first read about this study, I thought, *That's not going to work. You have to change their whole diet, not just a few minerals and essential omega-3 oils.* But you can't make major changes in only one group's diet and still have a double-blind study. People will know if all of a sudden they are eating a different diet—fruits, whole grains, and vegetables, for example.

So the only difference between the diets of these two groups was mineral supplements and fish oil. The researchers found that after an average of 142 days, the young violent offenders who were receiving the real minerals and DHA/EPA oils were involved in 35 percent fewer violent and hostile acts than the group receiving the placebo.

The researchers were blown away. The results were far better than those of any anger management program that had been done. The results were better than those achieved by any type of rehabilitation program. "Maybe," they said, "we should be paying attention to what we feed our prisoners. Maybe we should be paying attention to what we feed those young people who are at the greatest risk of ending up in prison." This powerful study showed that even a small amount of the right minerals and the right nutrients can transform behavior.

CHOOSING TO AVOID STRESS

One element of the Hippocratic Oath, important to physicians, is "Do no harm." That's important, of course. But what about doing some good? What about focusing on the priority issues that actually help the body heal naturally?

What is in your exposome—the sum total of your life experiences— right now that is overriding and dominating your genetic expression? That's an important question you should be asking yourself. I ask myself these questions regularly:

>> What am I doing?

>> What am I exposed to?

>> What's in my environment?

>> What's in my food?

>> What is in my thought processes?

>> Am I allowing myself to become frustrated because I need to rush here or there?

Have you ever gotten behind a car that is going slower than you want to go? Of course you have. How do you react? Just remember, you're not in charge of that other person's driving or the fact that he or she is driving slower than you would like. And it's not their fault that you are late or in a hurry. Don't let it upset you. You can choose to stay calm. When in stressful situations, choosing a calm demeanor and a humble attitude can have a powerful effect on your genetic expression and dramatically affect your personal risk of disease and your potential for health and healing.

CAFFEINE AND ADRENAL FATIGUE

Is stress always a bad thing? Not necessarily. Stress can actually save your life. Show me somebody who has no stress whatsoever, and I'll show you a dead person. You can't be alive and not have some stress. The key is to learn how to respond appropriately to different types of stress. Not only is stress inevitable, you actually *need* a certain level of stress in order to be healthy. If you have lost your ability to release stress hormones adequately and optimally, you're not going to be healthy.

If you have low stress hormones all the time, you're going to feel horrible. You're going to be in severe fatigue. It's called adrenal fatigue. So you don't want a life without any stress. Instead, you want to learn how to manage and optimized stress in the right way. You want to master it, not destroy it. By destroying stress, you destroy your own health.

There is a lot of talk these days about the benefits of coffee, specifically the caffeine in coffee. The new take on coffee is everywhere—magazine articles, the Internet, TV news and talk shows. It all reflects a huge amount of work, and even research, that seems to imply that coffee and caffeine are good for you. The message is that if you're not drinking coffee, you're missing out on a very important wellness strategy. It that true?

ASSOCIATION, NOT CAUSE

There was a very large study conducted at Harvard University, involving some 42,000 men and about 84,000 women. So this wasn't a small, pilot study. This was a huge epidemiological study. Epidemiological studies, which are the typical type of research study, don't necessarily establish cause and effect. They show association. An extreme example will illustrate the difference.

Almost 100 percent of persons who have died of a heart attack have eaten carrots. In that sense, heart attacks and eating carrots are strongly associated events. But that association in no way establishes that eating carrots *causes* heart attacks. Association allows us to theorize a potential cause and effect; it doesn't establish a cause and effect relationship.

When I was in my professional training, one of the best textbooks I ever bought was a little booklet titled, *How to Lie With Statistics*. It's easy to spew out all kinds of accurate information and still totally mislead. The information is accurate, but the interpretation is where the deception can take place.

COFFEE—RISK OR BENEFIT?

Back to the Harvard study. It showed that those who drank six or more cups of coffee a day, were statistically *less* likely to develop diabetes over the next eight years. Women were 29 percent less likely, and men were 54 percent less likely.[8] Guess what corporations promoted that finding all over the media!

If I told you that I believe the statistics are valid, what would you do? Would you start drinking coffee as a way to lower your risk of diabetes or its complications? Well, I believe the study's findings; it's an accurate study. But the problem is in how most people interpret that information. The average person who hears that finding is going to think, *Wow! If I start drinking six plus cups of coffee a day, I could dramatically improve my health and maybe even prevent getting diabetes. But if I drank that much coffee a day, I'd be a mess! No one could stand to be around me. I can't do that. But if six or seven cups of coffee are good for you, even one or two must have some health value. So maybe I'll drink two or three cups of coffee a day and get some health benefit. I won't go to extremes.*

Here's the mistake in that approach. Studies show that people who drink one or two or three cups of coffee a day actually have a *higher* risk for prediabetes[9] and a *higher* risk for abnormal blood pressure.[10, 11] What? If that's true, how can people who drink six or more cups of coffee cups a day, have a *lower* risk?

Here is where we have to start using our frontal lobes and learn how to reason from cause to effect. Let's look at the clinical studies, the studies that actually give caffeine to people and then measure what occurs in their bodies. Guess what happens. Blood sugars shoot way up;[12] insulin resistance increases;[13] blood pressure shoots up; the heart starts beating faster.

Clinical studies can produce very different findings in contrast to studies that look at association across population groups.

But is there any benefit from drinking coffee or using caffeine? The short answer is—Yes, there is benefit. Why would people do it if there weren't any benefit? People who are used to drinking a cup or two of coffee or other caffeinated beverage, feel better when they drink it. It takes out the cobwebs and helps them focus on the day. It can give them a shot of energy. It can make them more relaxed and agreeable. It loosens them up. Studies show that caffeine is also a mild hypnotic agent. When someone drinks a cup of coffee, they become easier to persuade to your point of view.[14] So there are multiple potential benefits associated with drinking coffee.

The longer answer to the above question requires that we ask another very important question. We must ask, "What is the downside?" In other words, in the long term, when used daily for weeks, months, and years, is caffeine mainly a benefit or is it a risk to our health?

And why would a group of people drinking large amounts of coffee over eight years, have a lower risk of diabetes? Let me tell you why I think that could be true. I believe people who drink that much coffee have adrenal fatigue. They're not producing enough of the stress hormone. By drinking coffee, they're actually medicating their energy levels. People with adrenal fatigue are unable to consistently produce adequate cortisol throughout the day. Without optimal levels of the stress hormone, cortisol, a person is going to feel tired.

Coffee, with its high caffeine content, forces the weak, fatigued adrenal glands to produce more cortisol, thus helping these people to feel better temporarily. But there is a cost.

Caffeine is forcing the body to use up the energy reserves that should be there for tomorrow and the next week. Such habitual use of caffeine will, over many years, wear down the adrenal glands and steal energy and vitality from our future. It basically ages us prematurely.

Another factor to consider is that the studies that seem to suggest a health benefit from drinking coffee are statistically controlling for the negative effects of other unhealthful behaviors. For instance, when studying the health risk associated with coffee, the researchers first remove the negative effect of smoking. But there is a major problem with this approach, because drinking coffee dramatically increases the desire to smoke![15] If I've learned anything from studying lifestyle medicine, it is that we must always consider the multiple ways each of our choices has an impact on other more important choices that affect our health. Our health choices don't operate independently of each other. They each affect numerous factors. In the end we must make choices that have a high benefit-to-cost ratio and avoid those behaviors that might be beneficial in a single area, but which overall make us much less healthy.

It's the same idea with smokers. Smokers aren't smoking in order to feel better than non-smokers. They're smoking more and more, trying to feel almost as good as non-smokers! Every cigarette makes them feel better. But is there a cost? Absolutely! Smokers know that. But they also know that if they smoke a cigarette, there will be a short-term benefit. They will feel less stress; they'll feel better. But overall, compared to before they started smoking, they actually feel more stress and more anxiety even after another cigarette. We always need to consider the benefit/cost ratio. That's the challenge. There may be a five-minute benefit, but what is the cost to our health over the weeks, months, and years?

> The bottom line is that stimulants—caffeine, nicotine, etc.—are effective short-term solutions for stress and adrenal fatigue, but long term, they are a disaster to our health.

I've had many patients who have been a Type A, executive kind of person all their adult lives. They're getting things done from morning until night. They're drinking coffee all morning long to keep that high level of activity and production going. They keep that up for decades. And then they hit their mid-50s, or whenever it might be, and they crash. They literally hit the adrenal fatigue wall. They tell me, "I just can't do this anymore. I used to be able to work hard all the time." Their strategy for controlling stress and optimizing energy ended up being a strategy for tearing down the reserve capacity of their adrenal glands.

There is a great way to test for adrenal fatigue. When patients come into my office and tell me, "I'm just so tired. I have a hard time concentrating, and

I don't handle stress very well anymore," I often recommend, among other tests, a four-hour glucose tolerance test. Especially if they are feeling tired in the late morning or mid-afternoon. This test measures blood sugars after not eating since dinner the night before. Blood sugar is tested at 8:00 A.M., and then a glucola drink is given that contains 75 grams of glucose. Blood sugars are again taken after thirty minutes and also at one, two, three, and four hours after the sugar drink. Patients with adrenal fatigue can have either high or normal blood sugars initially, but they often show large drops in blood sugars later in the test. It's best also to test insulin blood levels at fasting (and again after one and two hours), and cortisol stress hormone blood levels at fasting and again at three and four hours into the glucose tolerance test. It's a great test to evaluate whether a person has prediabetes or diabetes. It shows whether you have high insulin levels which drive cardiovascular disease and cancer.[16] It shows whether your cortisol output is normal, high, or low. It tells if your adrenal glands have "gone offline" because they can't handle the stress load any more. It is a three-dimensional model of the body's hormonal regulation of metabolism, and it provides key insights into what's out of balance and what we need to do to restore health and vitality.

> We should be trying to figure out how to manage stress and feel better right now, but in a way that also allows us to feel better later on—and in a way that doesn't tear down our adrenal glands but builds them up so they can produce optimal cortisol levels as we need it.

The goal for a two-pack-a-day smoker shouldn't be just to stop smoking. The goal should be to find and implement a group of wellness strategies that will make him feel so much better that he won't have the need to smoke anymore. That's the only way he is really going to be successful. Otherwise, even if he quits, he is just going to be a miserable, unhealthy non-smoker. We have to find a positive solution that takes the place of the dysfunctional one.

Chronic disease and health dysfunction is mostly caused by a deficiency of some kind—a missing wellness strategy or a lack of nourishment. Adrenal fatigue is often initiated or aggravated by poor digestion, which then leads to inadequate nutritional nourishment of the body systems. So to effectively manage stress we first need to make sure that we're taking advantage of optimizing digestion. In fact, one of the challenges with caffeine is that it impairs digestion. It impairs the body's ability to absorb minerals into the system.[17] It causes your kidneys to flush out critical amounts of many minerals, especially magnesium and calcium.[18]

> With caffeine we get the worst of both worlds. First, we absorb fewer minerals from our diet, and then we excrete more of them through our kidneys and urine.

With 75 percent of Americans not getting even the recommended intake of magnesium,[19] it's no wonder that very few of us have healthful levels of magnesium circulating in our bloodstream.

STRESS AND A REGULAR SCHEDULE

The body likes to be on a regular schedule. I'm not talking about being rigid. I'm talking about following a balanced and timely schedule—give or take thirty minutes. I'm talking about going to bed at a fairly consistent time most nights and getting up at generally the same time most mornings. Few things de-stress us better than getting outside in the sunlight for thirty minutes each morning. Do we regularly eat breakfast and lunch? Eating a light, early evening meal, or none at all, is a great strategy to improve your metabolism, especially if you are trying to lose weight, lower blood sugars, blood fats, or blood pressure. It's important to find a balance and work on a schedule that you know will be good for your body. Not following a reasonably predictable schedule is very stressful to our genes. When our body systems are in sync with bedtime, wake time, mealtime, and bright-light time, our genes will then be able to properly anticipate what is coming next. This will help ensure that our "good" genes are turned on and that our "bad" genes are turned off. The body likes to know when you're going to be waking up, or eating, or going to bed. And when you don't follow that general schedule, the body gets stressed. One reason everyone is under so much stress today is that we're not paying attention to the circadian rhythm, the natural light/dark cycle, the timeliness, and the chronobiology of health. Artificial lighting and round-the-clock schedules have thrown our bodies off kilter and increased our stress levels.

However, life and wellness aren't just about following a list. They're about understanding. They're about recognizing all the factors that influence your health in powerful ways. As you look at your life, can you identify stress factors? Can you think of ways to minimize harmful stress in your life? What changes can you make this week, this month, that will help "stress-proof" your life?

Based on what we have discussed in this chapter, what are some things that you should limit or take out of your life? What should you add to your life? How can you optimize who you can become—physically, emotionally, socially, and spiritually? There is an intimate relationship between all these aspects of your life. What you do in your social life, what you do for your physical health, how you interact emotionally, what's going on spiritually—all these things are interrelated. They all influence each other. How you respond to stress in one area affects all the other areas. The good news is that removing an unhealthful stress from just one aspect of your life will help bring about an overall improvement in many other parts of your life as well. Take a moment right now to make that short list. What will you limit? What will you add? Can you start acting on that list today? Why not right now?

CHAPTER SUMMARY

» There is a close connection between the body and the mind. What affects one also affects the other.

» Passive stress is bad for your health; active stress can be good for you. When you have a health problem, just waiting to see what happens causes passive stress. Active stress is taking steps to understand the problem and do whatever you can to improve it.

» Stress management techniques can actually "turn on" disease-preventing genes and "turn off" genes that promote disease.

» Stressful situations have the potential to dramatically increase blood sugars but can also cause unhealthful, low blood sugars.

» A four-hour Glucose Tolerance Test is a great way to evaluate your tendency to both high and low blood sugars and whether your adrenal glands are stressed or fatigued.

» Restoring the inner self through mental, spiritual, and physical rejuvenation enhances vitality and health.

» Stimulants such as caffeine and nicotine are effective short-term solutions for stress and adrenal fatigue, but with regular use over months and years, they are a disaster to your physical and emotional health.

» A regular, balanced schedule for eating, sleeping, and other activities reduces stress and promotes overall health.

ENDNOTES

1 Ellen White, *The Ministry of Healing*, p. 241.

2 Ibid.

3 Richardson, R., "Affective Style and *In Vivo* Immune Response: Neurobehavioral Mechanisms," *Proceedings for the National Academy of Sciences*, September 16, 2003; 100(19): 11148-11152.

4 Ornish, D., "Changes in Prostate Gene Expression in Men Undergoing an Intensive Nutrition and Lifestyle Intervention," *Proceedings of the National Academy of Sciences*, June 17, 2008; vol. 105, no. 24; 8369–8374.

5 Spiegel D., "Effect of Psychosocial Treatment on Survival of Patients with Metastatic Breast Cancer," *Lancet*, October 14, 1989; 2(8668):888-891.

6 Ezekiel 1:26.

7 Gesch, C., "Influence of Supplementary Vitamins, Minerals and Essential Fatty Acids on the Antisocial Behaviour of Young Adult Prisoners: Randomised, Placebo-Controlled Trial," *British Journal of Psychiatry*, (2002): 181, 22-28.

8 Salazar-Martinez, E., "Coffee Consumption and Risk for Type 2 Diabetes Mellitus," *Annals of Internal Medicine*, January 6, 2004;140(1):1–8.

9 Mos, Lucio, of San Antonio Hospital at the University of Padova, Italy, "HARVEST (Hypertension and Ambulatory Recording Venetia STudy)," reported at the annual meetings of the European Society of Cardiology, Sepember 2, 2014.

10 Zhang, Z., "Habitual Coffee Consumption and Risk of Hypertension: a Systematic Review and Meta-Analysis of Prospective Observational Studies," *American Journal of Clinical Nutrition*, June, 2011; vol. 93, no. 6, 1212-1219.

11 Palatini, P., "CYP1A2 Genotype Modifies the Association Between Coffee Intake and the Risk of Hypertension," *Journal of Hypertension*, (2009): 27(8):1594–1601.

12 Lane, J., "Caffeine Impairs Glucose Metabolism in Type 2 Diabetes," *Diabetes Care*, August, 2004; vol. 27, no. 8; 2047-2048.

13 Keijzers, G., "Caffeine Can Decrease Insulin Sensitivity in Humans," *Diabetes Care*, (2002): 25:364–369.

14 Martin, P., "Caffeine, Cognition, and Persuasion: Evidence for Caffeine Increasing the Systematic Processing of Persuasive Messages," *Journal of Applied Social Psychology*, January, 2005; vol. 35, issue 1; 160–182.

15 Shoaib, M., "Chronic Caffeine Exposure Potentiates Nicotine Self-Administration in Rats," *Psychopharmacology*, March, 1999; 142(4):327-333.

16 Giovannucci, E., "The Role of Insulin Resistance and Hyperinsulinemia in Cancer Causation," *Current Medicinal Chemistry*, 5 (2005): 53-60.

17 Bohn, T., "Dietary Factors Influencing Magnesium Absorption in Humans," *Current Nutrition & Food Science*, (2008); 4:53-72.

18 Kynast–Gales, S., "Effect of Caffeine on Circadian Excretion of Urinary Calcium and Magnesium," *Journal of the American College of Nutrition*, vol. 13, issue 5, 1994.

19 World Health Organization, "Calcium and Magnesium in Drinking Water: Public Health Significance," (Geneva: World Health Organization Press; 2009).

—SEVEN—

Positively Healthy

Attitudes and Healing

THROUGHOUT THIS BOOK, WE'VE FOCUSED ON THE EXPOSOME—
all the different things in our lives that change the way our genes work. The things that change the expression of our genes. The genes themselves don't change, but it isn't our genes that primarily determine our risk to various diseases or health issues. It's the expression of those genes, whether they have been activated, turned on or off, that determines our health risks.

All the factors in the exposome influence our genes, but some have a much greater impact than others. There is a whole field of study, *nutrigenomics*, that looks at how the food we eat influences our genetic risk. The power of food to alter genetic expression is significant and well documented. But in terms of affecting our genetic risk, there is something even more powerful than what we choose to put in our mouths. I'm referring to our emotions, moods, and mental attitudes. I believe that addressing this aspect of our exposome has a much greater potential to lead to healing than does optimizing our diet. Ironically, improving our diet is one of the ways to significantly improve our attitudes and emotions.[1]

THE HEALTH RISKS OF BEING A JERK

When someone cuts you off in traffic what is your instinctive response? Do you think, *That person is obviously in more of a hurry than I am. Probably late for something important. I'm going to slow down a little and let him go ahead?* Or do you get upset and angry that he had the nerve to cut you off?

Your reaction is part of your exposome!

About twenty-five years ago I was commuting three days a week between Loma Linda, California, and San Diego. Back then it was an eighty-five-mile drive. Traffic on the Southern California freeways then wasn't the nightmare it is today, but even so there were long delays, especially in construction areas where several lanes would narrow down to only one. When this happened, cars would be backed up for miles. And, of course, there were always drivers who would pull out of line and drive down the lane that was closing, past all the waiting cars, until they had to try to cut back in.

One afternoon, in frustration, I vowed that no one was going to cut in ahead of me. I wasn't going to let this bad behavior continue! A woman in the closed lane reached the point she had to stop and try to get back in line. She was right beside me. I deliberately moved my car up close to the one in front so she couldn't get in.

I gestured toward her with my arms open, as if to say, "What's your problem? You're not getting in here!" Just then, I looked over at her, and she looked over at me—and immediately I recognized her! She had been a classmate in my biochemistry class five years earlier!

I could have let her in. I could have shown her with some body language that I was sorry and then made room for her to get in line. But I had been fuming about the traffic for so long and it all happened so quickly that I just turned my gaze forward and didn't look back at her again.

That incident haunts me still. I've forgotten her name. I'd love to go back and ask her to forgive me for being such a jerk. I'm sure that's how she has thought of me for the past twenty-five years!

We laugh about such experiences, and we've all had them. One misdeed doesn't necessarily establish a pattern. But sometimes there are other experiences in our lives that are much more serious and have long lasting implications for one's health. What about the experiences that bring about bitterness and resentment? How do they affect our epigenome? How do such attitudes affect our health?

CAN ATTITUDES REALLY AFFECT HEALING?

Can our attitudes actually affect our health and healing?

I'd like to suggest to you that our attitudes have a *huge* impact on healing and that if we don't address negative attitudes, we're not going to come close to achieving our healing potential, now or in the future.

> As we become more self-aware, we realize that we need healing in many areas of our lives—physically, emotionally, and spiritually. And our attitudes and emotions play a major role in bringing about the healing we all need.

Is it possible that while we are following a wellness program, exercising daily, eating a wholesome, healthful diet, spending time in the sunlight—doing everything we know to do to optimize our health—we can still be missing the most important wellness strategy of all by overlooking the influence of our mental outlook on our health?

SURVEYING YOUR ATTITUDES

Nancy was in her early 60s when she first came to see me some years ago. She had been a school teacher all her adult life, and now that she was getting close to retirement age, she was looking forward to traveling and doing fun things. She wanted to enjoy optimal health in her retirement years, so she joined a comprehensive lifestyle medicine program.

Within two weeks of beginning the program, she had reversed her high blood pressure. Her prediabetes was reversed within a month. She was ecstatic about how much better she was feeling and that so many areas of her health were improving. She came to realize that the program wasn't just about getting blood sugars and cholesterol under control. It was more than just controlling weight and blood pressure. It was more even than exercise and diet. Nancy came to understand that the program involved looking at every factor, every aspect of the exposome, that has an influence on health and wellness.

About halfway through the six-month program, I gave Nancy's group a survey found in the book, *Anger Kills,* by Dr. Redford Williams and his wife, Dr. Virginia Williams. Dr. Redford Williams, a well-known psychiatrist, was the director of the Behavioral Medicine Center at the University of North Carolina. In the twenty years that I've been using this forty-six-question survey with my patients, I've seen it help many of them to become significantly more self-aware about their attitudes and the influence these have on health and healing.

The survey is actually measuring hostility. Each question sets up a scenario and asks you to choose one of two responses. You might like to have a third choice, but you have to choose between the two responses given. When I first took the survey years ago, I didn't think I was very hostile in my attitudes. In high school, I was always seen as the peacemaker when friends would become angry with each other. But the survey helps you see that hostility is not manifested only in physically aggressive acts or in threatening or intimidating behavior. Hostility includes the emotion of anger. It doesn't stop there. Most of us don't realize that hostility can be as subtle as a mental attitude.

Hostility also involves what we're thinking. An attitude of mistrust or cynicism is actually the most common form of hostility.

Of course, there is much that is wrong with the world we live in. When we look at the political climate, the economic situation, society, it's easy to be cynical and angry. The challenge is to not let these things become part of our daily exposome, because our attitudes shape us at the genetic level. We have to learn to become masters of our genes even at the level of our attitudes.

As Nancy and her group were answering the questions on this survey, I was watching their reactions. I'd gotten to know these people well over the past three months. We'd talked together about intimate goals and concerns. I could see them becoming more self-aware regarding their attitudes. They were realizing that there is more going on that affects their health than just the exercise program or what they eat.

After everyone had finished the survey, we discussed the issues it raised. People began asking questions. "How can we deal with hostility in our daily lives?" "How can we witness wrongs and injustice and yet not let anger and cynicism take over our thinking?" "How can we live in peace with our neighbors and friends and families?" So I challenged the group to come up with specific suggestion for things they could do in the next twenty-four hours to address these concerns.

"GET OUT OF MY HOUSE!"

At the end of the session, Nancy came to me. She had been crying a little. She realized that she had been overlooking the most important thing in her wellness program.

Could that be true of you as well? Are conflict and negative attitudes ongoing risk factors in your epigenome?

Nancy began sharing her experience with me, letting me know why this hostility questionnaire was hitting so close to home for her.

"Twenty years ago," she said, "my best friend and I bought homes right next to each other. We did everything together. We had decided that we were going to raise our children together. Then one evening we were playing games and talking, when my friend said something about my son that offended me so much that I looked at her and said, 'Get out of my house! I don't ever want to see you again!'

"She stared at me and said, 'I'm sorry! I wasn't thinking.'

"'Get out of my house,' I repeated.

"We still live next door to each other, but I haven't talked to her in twenty years. If I happen to go outside for some reason and see her, I turn away. I don't want to see her. I don't want to deal with her. She does the same. Once in a while we will happen to drive in at the same time. We get out of our cars and walk into our houses without looking at each other. We keep the blinds closed on the windows that face each other. We don't want any reminders that we used to be friends."

Then Nancy looked at me and said, "I've just realized what a horrible, terrible mistake I've made. What do I do now?"

We talked about the situation, and we prayed together. I told her, "Nancy, I want you to think about what you can do in the next twenty-four hours to address that conflict."

You see, this conflict in Nancy's life wasn't just something that had happened twenty years ago. It was an ongoing conflict that she had been experiencing every day for the past twenty years. It needed to be resolved. If it wasn't cleaned up and taken care of, it would gradually destroy her.

> This conflict was the number one risk factor endangering her health. That emotional conflict was far more important than controlling her prediabetes or her high blood pressure. It was far more important to her health than her weight or her cholesterol or anything else. These negative attitudes were stressing her out and eating her up inside.

HOSTILITY AND HEALTH

Are you going through some conflict like that? If so, how is it affecting your genetic expression? How is it changing your current health and your risks for the future? These issues are part of a new scientific discipline called psycho-neuro-endocrine genomics, or psycho- neuro-endocrine immunology, that is looking at the way genes work and the influence our attitudes have on them. We are learning more about the effect of our minds and how we think on our nervous system. The nervous system, in turn, influences our hormonal system, and those hormones position the immune system to respond in one way or another. Ultimately, all of this influences our genes—expressing our gene function in the direction of either healing or disease.

In a study done at the University of North Carolina researchers gave medical students who were in their final year of training the Minnesota Multiphasic Personality Inventory. The forty-six questions that Dr. Redford Williams put into his book, *Anger Kills,*[2] are part of that comprehensive inventory. I recommend you read that book, especially if you discover that you're one of the 20 percent of individuals who are "hot reactors." Hot reactors don't find it easy to shrug things off. They are easily offended and upset. They hang on to resentment and bitterness.

There are ways of dealing with these issues, just as there are with all other health risks. If you're a hot reactor, it doesn't mean you're not a good person. It just means that you need to understand yourself and the risk factors you're facing and find ways to deal with them. Being honest with yourself and being accountable to a process of change will ultimately bring happiness and joy back into your life along with vibrant health.

In the University of North Carolina study, these young student physicians, most of whom were around 25 years old, took this comprehensive personality inventory. The study then followed these individuals over a period of decades. It found that those who scored in the upper half of their class for hostility were five times more likely to develop heart disease by age 50 than those who scored lowest for hostility! That is a 500 percent greater risk! They were also seven times more likely to have died by age 50 from all causes combined.[3] These kinds of risk factors don't show up very often. These are huge risk factors.

Researchers from the Mayo Clinic found that hostility speeds progression of heart disease and dramatically increases the risk of a heart attack at a younger age.

In fact, "the prevalence of hostility symptoms was 3.5 times higher in young patients (28 percent vs. 8 percent). Young patients with hostility symptoms also had more adverse CAD (coronary artery disease) risk profiles, including higher total cholesterol levels, triglycerides levels, total cholesterol/high-density lipoprotein cholesterol ratios, fasting glucose levels and glycosylated hemoglobin levels, and lower quality-of-life scores compared with young patients with low hostility scores." Having emotional anger, a mistrusting approach to life, harboring frustration inside—these things dramatically increase the risk of heart disease. The good news is that simply participating in a twelve-week cardiac rehabilitation and exercise training program led to "marked improvements in CAD risk factors, behavioral characteristics (including hostility), and quality of life—and a nearly 50 percent reduction in the prevalence of hostility symptoms."[4][5]

The University of North Carolina also looked at law students and found similar results. In a group of law students who were given the comprehensive personality inventory at age 25, those who scored highest for hostility experienced high mortality rates. By age 50, 20 percent of them had died, compared with only 4 percent of those scoring low for hostility!

> There is a profound statement made by King Solomon. Speaking of our human nature, he states: "As . . . [a man] thinks in his heart, so is he."[6] That is not only a powerful spiritual principle, it's also a psychological principle and a physiological principle.

In the human brain there is a neuropeptide called proopiomelanocortin— or POMC, for short. POMC is a protein whose chemical structure is such that it can be broken down into different molecules depending on where its coiled, amino acid chain is cleaved or split.[7, 8] If it is split on one side, it releases a new chemical that gives us a sense of joy and pleasure. This is where endorphins, the enkaphalins, come from. These endorphins are responsible for the high that runners get, that amazing feeling of accomplishment, that rush of energy and second wind. But if the POMC protein chain is split on the opposite side, it leads to the release of stress hormones that can make you anxious, stressed, depressed, and sad.

What makes the difference? How can this very same neuropeptide cause joy and pleasure on the one hand or sadness, despondency, and stress on the other? I'd like to suggest that it's a matter of our spirit. What attitude do we bring to the table? What attitude do we bring to situations in which someone has offended us or belittled us or has said something hurtful to us? What attitude do we exhibit when we are talking and interacting with others?

ATTITUDE IS A CHOICE

The thoughts and attitudes we dwell on and the way we respond to situations are, in fact, choices. We can choose how our minds and our bodies respond to various stimuli. We need to learn to allow the frontal lobe of our brain to be in control of our attitudes and responses. We need to reason from cause to effect and recognize that if we choose to respond in a spirit of vengeance, a spirit of bitterness, there will be negative consequences. We need to consider how that is going to affect us now and long term, as well as the effect our attitude has on those around us. A negative attitude is a real risk factor for diminishing our health and wellness. How we think, our attitudes, change the expression of our genes. You could say that our genes recognize our mental attitudes and react accordingly—either positively or negatively.

Those who struggle with hostility issues often rationalize their attitude by insisting, "That's just the way I am, and people need to accept it." It may be true that some people have a personality that is more prone to anger or hostility or aggression. But excusing it by saying, "That's just the way I am," doesn't allow for any effective or beneficial change to occur. We don't have to accept something that is hurtful to us and others. Why not seek to change our attitude into one that is more positive? There are ways to do that.

> One of the first things that you can do if you discover that you have cynicism, anger, or hostility in your life is to change your diet.

Changes to your diet can make it easier to control hostility, but you still must choose how you are going to respond to various situations. You can be on the very best diet in the world, but if you continue to make poor choices regarding your responses, your attitudes, in different situations, you're still going to affect your health negatively. More than forty-five studies have shown that hostility and physical health are strongly influenced by each other.[9, 10] Hostility is a risk factor for heart disease, premature death, and a wide spectrum of health problems.[11]

You're much more likely to have a heart attack when you're angry or upset. Anger causes blood to coagulate.[12] The platelets in the blood begin to stick together, blood pressure climbs, the arteries contract, and if you have plaque buildup inside those arteries, this plaque can rupture, forming a clot. The result is a heart attack or stroke. Anger and tension precipitate all kinds of acute risk factors.

THE ZONE OF RUMINATION

A great many people are going about their daily routines carrying a seed of resentment or bitterness toward something or someone because of a hurtful incident in the past. The seething feeling of frustration and resentment is always there in the background. One of my professors at Loma Linda University called this the "Zone of Rumination."

Cows and other ruminants eat some grass, chew it for awhile, swallow it, and just sit there. Then they bring the chewed grass back up and chew it some more. And swallow. And chew. And swallow. That's why they're called ruminants. They work their food over and over. If you have a sensitive stomach, you probably wouldn't want to watch animals ruminate. Especially if you are eating!

But we do that all the time with our emotions. We ruminate about them. We chew them over in our minds and push them down into our subconscious. And then we dredge them back up and chew over them some more. They're always there in the background. The bitterness and anger and resentment go on and on. The conflict is never resolved, and the zone of rumination grows and grows.

All this greatly increases our risk factors for disease and poor health. But there is a silver lining to be found even in this. Because if bitterness is tearing down our health, then resolving that bitter conflict will relieve the burden of chemical stress on our bodies and dramatically increase our potential for optimizing our health.

GUM CLUB

What happens in the mind can have an amazing effect on the body.

A woman was coming to my twelve-week seminar on reversing diabetes. She was a very brittle Type 1 diabetic. Her blood sugars were frequently in the 400-450 range. We were trying to get her blood sugars under 140 two hours after eating and around 110 before meals. She was far from these numbers and at high risk for kidney failure, blindness, retinal detachment, and possible amputations later in life.

As we went through the twelve-week series, her blood sugars improved significantly. She was exercising and dealing with her diet. She was getting out in the sunlight in the mornings and taking the right amount of insulin before meals. In short, she was trying to do everything right. She reached the point that her blood sugar levels were on target at least 90 percent of the time.

During one of the last sessions of the series, we discussed stress and the impact in has on blood sugar. A few weeks later, I met this woman in the hallway of the clinic. She stopped me and said, "I know you're busy, but you have to listen to what happened to me."

She told me that about a week earlier she was at home starting to prepare for dinner and had checked her blood sugar. For a Type 1 diabetic, it was perfect. About four hours after eating lunch, her blood sugar was 107. Just then her 12-year-old daughter walked in the door from school. She seemed upset; she wouldn't make eye contact with her mother.

"What's wrong?" the woman asked.

"Something happened at school today. I don't want to talk about it right now."

"Please tell me. Tell me what happened."

"I don't want to talk about it," the girl repeated. "I've got a softball game. Can you just take me to the softball game?"

So the mother and daughter drove to the softball park. The woman could tell her daughter was upset. She tried again to find out why.

"Can I just wait to talk until after the softball game?"

"Okay, honey."

After the game had been going on a few minutes, the woman suddenly remembered a conversation she had had with another parent whose daughter attended the same middle school. This parent had told her that some of the mothers were concerned that one of the male teachers seemed overly friendly with the girls in his classes. She hadn't paid much attention, but now it took on a lot more significance. Could something have happened between this teacher and her daughter?

She began talking to some of her daughter's friends who were watching the game. She asked them, "Did something happen at school today?"

"No. Nothing unusual happened."

"Did my daughter get in trouble at school?"

"No. We were with her the whole day. Nothing happened."

She began thinking that, of course, no one would know if something had happened behind closed doors. Her imagination was running away with her. An hour and a half later, when the game was over and her daughter was coming off the field, the woman was beside herself.

"Honey," she insisted, "you've got to tell me what happened!"

The daughter looked at her and said, "I knew you would get upset."

"I won't get upset; I just need to know what happened."

The daughter began crying. Her mother's heart was pounding. "What happened today at school?" She was trying not to shout.

"I got put on gum club," her daughter cried.

"Gum club? What is gum club?"

"I got caught chewing gum, and the teacher made me go around and pull gum out from underneath the desks. I was so embarrassed, and I knew you'd be upset!"

"Honey, I'm not upset that you got put on gum club. I'm upset, because you let me think something really bad had happened." She hugged her daughter. "It's okay. Just don't chew gum again in class."

Then the woman realized that she had been under high stress for a couple of hours. She went home and checked her blood sugar. It was 457! Without having one bite of food after lunch, her blood sugars had increased from 107 to 457 simply because of what had been going on in her mind for the past two hours.

PRINCIPLES TO PRACTICE

What goes on in our mind, whether it's a thought, a concern, or an attitude, has a huge impact on our body physiology and ultimately on our genetic expression.

> One of the principles we can put into practice to lower our risk of disease and optimize our health is to make sure that we don't let our emotions get the best of us.

One of our jobs as parents, spouses, friends, and colleagues is to model a behavior of gentleness even if someone is treating us poorly or inappropriately. A kind, gentle attitude defuses anger and allows healing and bonding to take place. Harboring anger or resentment against someone allows that person to live rent free inside your mind and to control your attitude.

There is another principle we can follow—the investment principle—that will help us control our thoughts and attitudes. I'm indebted to the insightful Christian writer, C. S. Lewis, for this principle. All of us know certain people that we don't like being around. Our tendency is to avoid them. But if, instead, we will invest ourselves emotionally in them, something wonderful happens. We start to like them! Why? Because we've invested something of ourselves in them. It's a psychological principle that when we say a kind word or we smile at a person who has offended us or whom we don't like, our attitude begins to change. We start appreciating that person. We begin to see them in the same way that God sees them, and that changes everything. It's the principle of investment.

EMOTIONAL ISOLATION AS A RISK FACTOR

Writing about the power our emotions and attitudes have on our overall health, Dr. Dean Ornish writes in his book, *Love and Survival*,[13] that feeling isolated or rejected leads to a two-fold or even three-fold greater risk of premature death from all causes. Health-wise, one of the greatest risk factors confronting us today is a feeling of isolation from other people. So many of us haven't tried to reach out and build connections with our neighbors, co-workers, fellow church members, or any kind of group.

> Human beings have a need to feel that they belong, that they have some kind of connection to other people. Otherwise, feelings of rejection set in, and that is a major risk factor for illness and poor health.

Dr. Ornish goes on to demonstrate from studies that feeling isolated or rejected is a more powerful predictor of poor health and decreased lifespan even than smoking, alcohol use, lack of exercise, or overeating! You may be doing a great job of avoiding all these commonly recognized risk factors for disease and poor health, but if you're not addressing your feelings, emotions, and mental attitudes, you're ignoring one of the most significant factors affecting your health.

EMOTIONAL DEFICIENCIES

Pain, dysfunction, and guilt build in our lives due to deficiencies. And remember there are all kinds of deficiencies. It isn't only a deficiency of minerals and essential oils or a deficiency of vitamins or a deficiency of fiber and colorful, whole-plant foods that cause health problems for our bodies. We need to fill our hearts and our minds with those things that most powerfully change our genetic expression. That means that we need to fill our minds with the opposite of hostility. And what is the opposite of hostility? Love and forgiveness.

When love and forgiveness increase, hostility automatically decreases. When hostility increases, love and forgiveness decrease. This is not just someone's idea of how life should work; Dr. Ornish is referring to a physiological study of the effect of our attitudes on our bodies. The overwhelming evidence in the scientific medical literature is that the answer to the number one risk factor that affects our health is learning to be good at forgiveness[14]—finding excuses to forgive people.[15]

> Forgiveness isn't easy. You can't give what you don't have. So if you don't feel like you have forgiveness, it's very difficult to give it to somebody else. There will always be conflicts in life, but the question is: "How do I deal with them? Am I eager to quickly resolve them?"

Henry Ford said that the secret to success is understanding other people's point of view. That can be a challenge sometimes! But if we're willing to be open-minded and try to look at life from another's perspective, we'll often find conflicts being resolved and broken relationships healed.

A FORGIVING SPIRIT CAN CHANGE YOUR LIFE

H. M. S Richards, Sr. was an amazing preacher whose ministry spanned much of the twentieth century. He had gone through some experiences dealing with religious institutions that made him extremely bitter. A prominent administrator in his church had been instrumental in creating policies that caused Richards' mother to lose her job. He had made some hurtful and unfair statements regarding the situation. Richards, who was in college at the time, seethed with anger and resentment against this church leader.

Years later, Pastor Richards realized that even though he had often preached about the value of forgiveness, he had never, himself, forgiven this man. He had allowed his resentment regarding this issue to become part of his zone of rumination. The unfairness had continued to stir up and agitate negative emotions in his heart.

When he finally realized what has happening in his own life and acknowledged his need to forgive this individual, he found out where the man was living. It was a retirement home. No one ever came to visit him. He was in the last year of his life and miserable. Pastor Richards introduced himself. The older man remembered him and his parents. Richards went on to explain how upset he had been when the unfortunate incident had happened and how bitter and resentful he had continued to be throughout the years that had passed since then. The former church official told Richards that he understood. He understood why Richards would feel that way.

Then Pastor Richards said, "I want you to know that I forgive you. I forgive you, because I want to completely wipe the slate clean. I don't want to have any resentment in my life toward anyone."

Richards' act of forgiveness and the other man's acceptance of that forgiveness ended in a friendship. For the last year of this man's life, Pastor Richards was one of the few people who regularly visited him at the retirement home, giving them both a sense of joy and a new understanding of what it means to be forgiven.

> When we forgive someone who has deeply wronged us, we have an opportunity to change that person's life, but we also dramatically change our own.

You see, we're not responsible for how others may respond to our forgiveness. We can't control that. But we can forgive. We can control our own feelings and resolve the conflict in our own minds.

There are always going to be times and situations in life when conflict arises. You will have to deal with people who have a different perspective than you do—different goals and ideas that conflict with yours. How you handle these situations has a great deal to do with your current and future health. Keeping a positive mental attitude is crucial.

As Seneca pointed out, "It is part of the cure to wish to be cured." Do you want to be healthy? The apostle Paul urges us not to follow the world's pattern but to be transformed by a renewal of our minds, a renewal of our mental attitudes.[16] Understanding the spiritual, emotional, and physical impact of forgiveness—and a willingness to forgive—will transform your relationships with others and your personal health.

One of my favorite promises in the book of Isaiah says, "Thou shalt be called, The repairer of the breach, The restorer of paths to dwell in."[17] Originally a promise to the Jewish people who after seventy years of exile in Babylon would rebuild the destroyed city of Jerusalem, these words are also a personal promise to each of us. It's a promise that we can repair broken relationships, that we can restore harmony and rest to our spirits.

When we are humble and willing to do what is right, it will revitalize the metabolic and genetic pathways that influence our health. A forgiving attitude is the only prescription, the only medicine, in the entire universe, powerful enough to unlock the chemical bonds of hostility, resentment, and bitterness that lock up our genes and prevent healing.

THE REST OF THE STORY

Let's go back to Nancy's story from early in this chapter. You'll remember that she hadn't spoken to her best friend in twenty years—her former very best friend. They had quarreled over an unthinking comment her friend had made.

"What can I do?" she asked me. "It's been twenty years; I can't just go up to her and tell her I'm sorry."

"Really?" I said. "It might be just that easy."

I could see the conflict in her heart and mind. "I'd feel like such a fool!"

That's just it, isn't it? If we want to be healthy, we must sometimes be willing to feel like a fool! So many things could go wrong. Her friend could laugh at her. She could hang up the phone. She could turn and walk away. What would Nancy do if any of those things happened? What would you do?

In the end, none of those things should be concerns. All Nancy could do was to try to resolve the misunderstanding. That's all you can do.

Nancy went home. About twenty minutes later, there was a knock at her door. It was her walking partner with whom she walked several times a day. Quickly, Nancy put on her walking shoes. She hadn't planned to walk right then; she was still distressed, trying to figure out how best to approach her former friend and heal this hurt between them. But she didn't want to disappoint her walking partner, so she went walking with her.

As they walked, Nancy couldn't help unburdening her heart. The partner didn't say anything; she just listened. As they finished exercising, Nancy exclaimed, "Thank you for listening; I still don't know what I'm going to do."

That night, Nancy tossed and turned. How was she going to approach her former friend? The next morning, there was a knock on the door. Nancy opened the door, and there was her walking partner, but standing right behind her was Nancy's former best friend! The two estranged women looked at each other—really looked at each other—for the first time in twenty years!

Overwhelmed with emotion, Nancy found herself taking the three steps off the porch to her driveway and walking toward her friend. Her friend met her and they threw their arms around each other.

"I'm so sorry," Nancy said, "for being so foolish, for being unwilling to ask for forgiveness."

"I'm the one who should have asked for forgiveness," her friend responded. "I'm sorry, Nancy."

They hugged and cried and then they went for a walk together—two women who had avoided each other for twenty years over a misunderstanding. Not just twenty wasted years, but twenty years of wearing, unending stress that was creating a terrible physiological risk factor for illness and disease.

What can you do—what *should* you do—today to resolve conflict and limit health risk in your life? As you learn about the vital role your mind plays in your physical health, you have the opportunity to take advantage of this new awareness. I challenge you to resolve any unresolved conflicts and cultivate a forgiving spirit. This is the most important thing you can do to bring true joy and health to your body, mind, and soul.

CHAPTER SUMMARY

>> Hostility is defined not just by aggressive actions and the emotion of anger, but also by the attitude of cynicism and distrust.

>> Improving our diet is a powerful and effective way to improve our attitudes and our overall emotional health.

>> Attitudes alter how our genes function and therefore greatly affect our potential for healing.

>> Attitude is a choice. Despite our temperament, we can choose how to respond to various situations.

>> What goes on in the mind has a huge impact on the body.

>> Emotional isolation is one of the most powerful predictors of poor health and decreased lifespan.

>> The opposite of hostility is forgiveness. As we experience receiving and giving forgiveness, hostility melts away.

>> A forgiving spirit can change your life.

>> We have all done things in our past that have hurt or damaged someone else. Why not ask for forgiveness?

>> If someone has hurt or damaged us, why not forgive them? Forgiveness doesn't remove the guilt of the offender. More important, it removes the ongoing trauma that unresolved hostility brings to our own body, mind, and soul.

>> The "Zone of Rumination" describes the seething feelings of frustration and resentment so many of us carry around with us as we continue to mull over some hurtful situation or individual from the past.

>> What can we do in the next twenty-four hours to bring resolution and closure to conflicts from our past?

ENDNOTES

1   Gesch, C. Bernard. "Influence of Supplementary Vitamins, Minerals and Essential Fatty Acids on the Antisocial Behaviour of Young Adult Prisoners," *British Journal of Psychiatry*, 181 (2002): 22-28.

2   Williams, Redford, and Williams, Virginia, *Anger Kills: 17 Strategies for Controlling the Hostility that Can Harm Your Health* (New York, NY: HarperCollins, 1994).

3   http://www.nytimes.com/1990/12/13/health/if-anger-ruins-your-day-it-can-shrink-your-life.html

4   Lavie, C., "Prevalence of Hostility in Young Coronary Artery Disease Patients and Effects of Cardiac Rehabilitation and Exercise Training", *Mayo Clinic Proceedings*, vol. 80, issue 3, 335–342.

5   "Reducing Hostility in Young Coronary Artery Disease Patients Is Important Piece Of Rehabilitation, Suggests Mayo Clinic Proceedings Study," *Science Daily*, April 8, 2005. <www.sciencedaily.com/releases/2005/03/050329131038.htm>

6   Proverbs 23:7, NKJV.

7   Raffin-Sanson, M.; de Keyzer, Y.; Bertagna, X., "Proopiomelanocortin, a Polypeptide Precursor with Multiple Functions: From Physiology to Pathological Conditions," *European Journal of Endocrinology* (2003) 149 (2): 79–90. doi:10.1530/eje.0.1490079. PMID 12887283.

8   Proopiomelanocortin (POMC) [*Homo sapiens* (human)] http://www.ncbi.nlm.nih.gov/gene/5443

9   Chida, Y., "The Association of Anger and Hostility with Future Coronary Heart Disease: A Meta-Analytic Review of Prospective Evidence," *Journal American College of Cardiology*, March 17, 2009; 53(11): 936-46. doi: 10.1016/j.jacc.2008.11.044.

10 Ford, K., "Review: Anger and Hostility Increase Risk of Coronary Heart Disease Events in Healthy People and Those with Existing CHD," *Evidence Based Nursing*, October 2009; 12(4):121. doi: 10.1136/ebn.12.4.121.

11 Niaura, Raymond; Banks, Sara M.; Ward, Kenneth D.; Stoney, Catherine M.; Spiro III, Avron; Aldwin, Carolyn M.; Landsberg, Lewis; and Weiss, Scott. T.; "Hostility and the Metabolic Syndrome in Older Males: The Normative Aging Study," in Cacioppo, John T.; et al, eds., *Foundations in Social Neuroscience*, (Cambridge, MA: MIT Press/Bradford Books, 2002), 1209–1223.

12 Von Känel, R., "Relation of Psychological Distress to the International Normalized Ratio in Patients with Venous Thromboembolism With and Without Oral Anticoagulant Therapy," *Journal of Thrombosis and Haemostasis*, August 2012; 10(8):1547-1555. doi: 10.1111/j.1538-7836.2012.04801.x.

13 Ornish, Dean, *Love and Survival* (New York: Harper Collins Publishers, 1998).

14 Lawler, Kathleen A.; Younger, Jarred W.; Piferi, Rachel L.; Jobe, Rebecca L.; Edmondson, Kimberley A.; and Jones, Warren H., "The Unique Effects of Forgiveness on Health: An Exploration of Pathways," *Journal of Behavioral Medicine*, 28, No. 2 (2005): 157–167.

15 McCullough, Michael E., and van Oyen Witvliet, Charlotte, "The Psychology of Forgiveness," in Snyder, C. R. and Lopez, S., eds., *Handbook of Positive Psychology*, (New York: Oxford University Press, 2002), 446-458.

16 See Romans 12:2.

17 Isaiah 58:12, KJV.

The New Normal
CHRONIC KIDNEY DISEASE

AMAZINGLY, AND WITHOUT MUCH FANFARE, WE HAVE now reached a point where the majority of Americans will suffer from chronic kidney disease in their lifetime. Yes, chronic kidney disease is the new normal. Now is the time to determine our personal risk and learn what we can do to prevent and reverse this condition.

About nine years ago, when I was living on the island of Guam, my neighbor, colleague, and friend, Dr. Hugo Leon, called me one Saturday afternoon. Dr. Leon is one of those people who is always helping someone in need. He has super high energy and is excited about life. He said, "Wes, can you come to the hospital right now?"

"I guess I could come," I answered. "What's up?"

He said, "I have a patient here, his name is John, who almost died last night, and he really wants to talk to you." Dr. Leon went on to explain that this 45-year-old fire-fighter had had diabetes for many years. The previous night he had come to the hospital, where he was diagnosed with acute kidney failure and had almost died. The next morning, family had come from all over the island to be with John, shocked that they had almost lost their son, their nephew, their father. They were all eager for him to get better.

A REASON TO HOPE

John realized that he had almost died and that he was now facing potential medical retirement. But he had heard Dr. Leon say something that gave him hope. The doctor had told him, "John, your diabetes is out of control; your blood pressure is out of control; your cholesterol is out of control; your overall health is out of control. But you can reverse all this if you really want to." He had never heard a doctor say this before. John was typical of many persons with chronic health complaints. He looked pretty fit on the outside—muscular, a fire-fighter. On the inside, however, he was rapidly dying. His blood sugars and his blood pressure were sky high, and he was increasingly developing other internal signs of disease.

I drove to the hospital that afternoon, and there was John. The nurse brought me John's chart. As I began reading it, I could see why he had ended up in the hospital and had almost died.

As a fire-fighter, John was used to dealing with emergencies. But in the down time between crises, he did what many fire-fighters do—he learned to cook tasty meals. Yes, he was aware that he had diabetes, but he hadn't really taken it seriously. He knew the statistics.

He knew that at least half of those between the ages of 40 and 59 already have prediabetes. He knew that two-thirds of those between 60 and 74 years of age are prediabetic and that three-fourths of those older than 74 are prediabetic and that a third have full-blown diabetes.[1]

So for John, having diabetes just seemed like part of the normal aging process. But he was only 45 years old.

As I looked at John's chart, I saw some alarming numbers. He weighed 229 pounds—not super heavy, but definitely overweight. His fasting blood sugar was 300 mg/dl; his random blood sugars two hours after meals were over 400 mg/dl; his cholesterol was 300. While cholesterol is often overemphasized as the key to heart disease, there is little question that John's very high cholesterol was placing him at significant risk. For instance, Dr. William Casteli, medical director of the Framingham Heart Study, wrote in the *American Journal of Cardiology* that after twenty-six years of follow up, study participants who had total cholesterol levels of 300 or higher were almost sure to get coronary heart disease. In fact, the likelihood of them being diagnosed with significant plaque buildup in their coronary arteries was 90 percent! Fortunately, only 3 percent of the American population have cholesterol levels that high.[2]

But, as we saw in Chapter 3, there are other tests that can further help us determine the actual risk for developing cardiovascular disease or other serious health complications. That is why it is so important to look at the broader picture, the advanced cardiovascular risk factors, so that we can truly pinpoint the underlying causes and do something about them—preferably before we end up in the hospital like John.

Even though John took two blood pressure medications, his blood pressure was still high at 150/100. His hemoglobin A1C level was at 16.6 percent—over three times higher than optimal. It was as if his blood was highly crystallized, given the amount of sugar that was glazing to his red blood cells and other tissues.

Yet, as I walked into John's room and looked into his face, I saw hope. Dr. Leon had told him, "You can change this situation. You don't have to go on with your life being at risk. You don't have to keep facing the danger that your body will shut down and die."

I could see in John's eyes that he was ready to make the necessary changes to become healthy. He told me, "I want to deal with this now. I want to do whatever it takes."

As we talked that Saturday afternoon in the hospital, John was beginning to understand that the issue wasn't just his blood sugar levels or his cholesterol numbers. The real issue was the underlying metabolic dysfunction from which all these problems stemmed. He could take more insulin to try to control his blood sugars. He could take more blood pressure medications—he was already on two. But doing all these things wouldn't be addressing the actual cause of the problem. John was beginning to understand that he had to focus on the basics, not on the superficial.

FOCUSING ON ROOT CAUSES

Other tests showed just how critical John's condition was. His creatinine level, a measure that indicates how well the kidneys are filtering toxins, stood at 5.8 when it should have been no higher than 1.2. This suggested to me that if doctors had not intervened immediately, John wouldn't have had many more hours to live.

We did a C-peptide test on John. This is a fundamental test for individuals who have diabetes and who are taking insulin. It is designed to determine whether the pancreas is still capable of producing adequate amounts of insulin on its own. John was taking more than 100 units of insulin each day. We needed to be able to determine why he needed that much insulin to lower his blood sugars. Was it because his pancreas wasn't making enough insulin or that his muscle and liver cells had become unresponsive to the insulin his body was making?

The C-peptide test showed us that John's pancreas was making plenty of insulin. A high C-peptide blood test strongly suggests that by introducing aggressive lifestyle medicine strategies, including exercise and dietary changes, there can be a dramatic reversal of the diabetes and its related complications.

Another complicating factor was that John had a very high level of potassium in his blood. His kidneys had essentially shut down and were no longer able to remove excess potassium. A high potassium level can lead to arrhythmias of the heart and fatal heart attacks. So John had been warned not to eat foods rich in potassium.

One of the challenges for people like John—people with serious medical conditions, especially advanced kidney problems—is that a first-class diet is vital if they are to become healthy.

If you are going to have first-class health, you have to eat first-class foods. These are the foods that are most nutrient-dense and that have the greatest potential to literally alter the environment around your genes and make positive changes in the way your genes work.

And one of the key components of a healthful diet is green, leafy vegetables. However, green leafy vegetables are also high in potassium.

Because of his high potassium levels, due to the fact that his kidneys had largely shut down and could not filter potassium out of his blood, John had been told not to eat green leafy vegetables. Legumes, another key food, are also very high in potassium. I call legumes the "king of foods" because of their amazing ability to help control soaring blood sugars, improve and lower cholesterol, and lower blood pressure. Legumes include beans, peas, and lentils. Ironically, it seemed that, because of his high potassium levels, John should not be eating the very kinds of food he actually needed in order to bring healing to his body! What was he to do?

Clearly, John needed to pay attention to the risks. He didn't want to aggravate his already high potassium level. But he was committed to a healthful lifestyle.

How did we solve the diet versus potassium problem?

As I talked with John's internist, we came up with a plan that worked. We had John take a prescription syrup, called Kayexalate, every day. This syrup binds to potassium in the gut, so that while John was eating all those healthy, high potassium foods, this Kayexalate syrup was able to bind to the excess potassium in the gut and remove it so that his blood potassium levels would not become so elevated that they posed a risk to his heart. This made it possible for John to eat the healthful, high-potassium foods he needed, without raising his potassium blood levels.

The amazing thing was that after just ten days in our wellness program, John no longer needed the Kayexalate. Because of the lifestyle and diet changes he had made, his kidneys had healed enough that they were able to function adequately and now keep his potassium at normal levels without the need for medication.

Within ten days of making these lifestyle changes, John was also able to quit taking insulin completely!

Within two weeks, he was completely off all his blood pressure medications! At this point, most of his blood sugars were under 110 fasting and under 130 two hours after meals. John was excited.

DRAMATIC TRANSFORMATIONS

Being a fire-fighter, John wasn't one to shrink from challenges. He was determined to protect his health and his family. As soon as he was released from the hospital, he began our lifestyle medicine program. We did a baseline evaluation at the beginning of the program, and then we did follow-up labs two weeks later. We were checking blood sugars and blood pressures before and after exercise, as well as before and after eating. We had John on a 100 percent plant-based diet. John was doing everything he could to optimize health.

Within a month after beginning the program, John's blood sugars were consistently under control. His blood pressure had come down to 100/75. His hemoglobin A1C dropped from 16.6 to 12.2 and kept dropping each month thereafter. By any standard, a hemoglobin A1C of 16.6 is out-of-control diabetes, and each point above 6 represents a 37 percent increased risk of kidney failure, blindness, and other complications.[3] So even at 12.2 John continued to have some serious risk. But as the numbers decreased week by week, his health continued to dramatically improve. The blood sugar problems in our body reverse very quickly if we are doing the right things.

Three months after entering the lifestyle medicine program, John's creatinine level had come down from a death defying 5.8 to 1.3, just slightly above the optimal range we like to see of 0.7 to 1.2. The level of microalbumin, protein lost in his urine, had dropped from 3,500 to 400 during those three months! His kidneys were still slightly damaged, but nowhere near as much as they had been during the first month after he almost died. John was now able to discontinue all his medications except for a low dose of a cholesterol lowering medicine which his internist continued as a preventive strategy because of his history of significant inflammation.

After just one week of being on an intensive lifestyle medicine program, John experienced a dramatic transformation. After ten days, he had reversed many of the risk factors he had been facing when he came into the hospital.

But his Cardiac CRP, the measure of systemic, whole-body inflammation, remained high throughout all these other amazing changes. I began looking for other factors that could possibly contribute to such elevated inflammation.

I went through the checklist of possible causes, and as I did so, I asked him to open his mouth. I'm not a dentist, but one look and I realized the cause of much of his systemic inflammation. Untreated dental problems such as gingivitis and periodontal disease are a significant source of inflammation and toxicity for your entire body[4] and specifically for kidney disease.[5] They are also a major factor in the risk of having a stroke or heart attack.[6]

Every time John went to the dentist, he was told it would cost thousands of dollars to fix the problems in his mouth. One dentist had given him the figure of fifteen thousand dollars!

I looked at him and said, "I understand, John. I wouldn't want to spend that much money either, but you almost died! You have to fix the underlying causes of your risk."

We know that inflammation turns on the diabetes genes.[7] Inflammation turns on and drives the cardiovascular disease genes and the cancer genes,[8] as well. But they also create havoc with the kidneys. John had almost died because of acute inflammatory kidney failure.

FOUR TESTS FOR KIDNEY HEALTH

I want to focus on four important tests we did with John and how they relate to the bigger issue of kidney health. The first is the **Glomerular Filtration Rate (GFR)**, which measures how well your kidneys are performing their basic function of filtering toxins from your body. The optimal range for the GFR test is 100 milliliters per minute or higher. That is the healthy rate at which your kidney should be filtering your blood and means the kidneys are functioning at 100 percent. A GFR of less than 90 is an early indication of sub-optimal kidney function.

TESTS TO EVALUATE KIDNEY FUNCTION

Test	Standard Levels	Optimal Levels
GFR or Glomerular Filtration Rate* When kidneys are functioning optimally, their filtration rate is high. When filtration rate drops, their ability to filter toxins decreases.	>60 mL/min.	>90 mL/min.
BUN (Blood Urea Nitrogen)* This test measures the amount of nitrogen in your blood that comes from the waste product urea. If your kidneys are compromised and are not able to properly remove urea from the blood, your BUN level rises.	9-28 mg/dL	9–20 mg/dL
Creatinine* This substance is generated from muscle metabolism. The kidneys should filter out most of the creatinine from your blood. An elevated creatinine level signifies impaired kidney function.	<1.5 mg/dL	<1.2 mg/dL
Microalbumin (Spot Urine Test) This test measures the amount of the protein albumin in your urine. If your kidneys are functioning properly, this level should be very low.	<30 mg/L	<20 mg/L

*These tests are all included in the Comprehensive Metabolic Panel (CMP). More information about these tests can be found at labtestsonline.org.

There are five stages of kidney disease, as shown in the chart above. Stage 3 chronic kidney disease begins when the GFR falls below 60 milliliters per minute. Ironically, Stage 3 kidney disease is so prevalent that often it is not even discussed during medical visits until the disease advances to Stage 4. Of course, our goal is to catch conditions early enough to prevent progression, but also to more easily reverse the condition completely.

The second test we looked at is the **Blood Urea Nitrogen (BUN)** test. Urea is the natural byproduct of protein metabolism in the body. If urea levels in the blood are elevated, we know that the kidneys are having a difficult time processing and filtering out this naturally occurring toxin in the body. Normal BUN levels should range from 7 to 25 mg/dL. One reason BUN levels may be elevated is that the person is dehydrated. So it is important to drink adequate amounts of

THE FIVE STAGES OF KIDNEY DISEASE

Stage	Description	GFR ml/min/1.73m^2
	Optimal Kidney Function	≥100
1(p)	Kidney damage with normal or raised eGFR	90-99
2(p)	Kidney Damage with mild decreased eGFR	60-89
3A(p)	Moderate decreased eGFR	45-59
3B(p)	Moderate decreased eGFR	30-44
4(p)	Severe decreased eGFR	15-29
5(p)	Kidney Failure	<15 or dialysis

water throughout the day as discussed in Chapter 5. Drinking only when you feel thirsty will not provide adequate hydration to optimize kidney function.

A third, very important, test measures the level of creatinine in the blood. Creatinine is generated from muscle metabolism. **The Creatinine test** is a key screening tool to evaluate how well the kidneys are filtering out these naturally occurring toxins. An elevated creatinine level signifies impaired kidney function. Optimal creatinine levels should be between 0.7 and 1.2 mg/dL.

The fourth test, the **Microalbumin Urine** test, looks at the amount of microalbumin in the urine. *Micro* means "small," and albumin is the most abundant protein in the blood. Even small amounts of protein found in the urine suggest the possibility of an early form of damage in the kidneys. In fact, albumin is the protein that helps draw fluid out of the tissues and back into the blood. So when people have swelling in their tissues, one of the main reasons is that albumin is not being filtered properly and is being dumped into the urine.

You want to keep the albumin and protein in the blood. If there are high levels (above 17 ug/ml) of microalbumin in the urine, that is a sign that the filtration process is damaged and is not able to hold onto this precious protein that the body has spent so much time and effort to build. The ratio of microalbumin to creatinine should be under 30.

REVERSING CHRONIC KIDNEY DISEASE

As noted above, there are five recognized stages of chronic kidney disease.[9] Frequently, I will see individuals with a kidney filtration rate (GFR) of less than 60, meaning that they are already at Stage 3A kidney disease and have already lost half their normal kidney function. When they hear this, they say, "What happened to stages one and two?" They haven't been aware of a problem until they are already progressing along the continuum of chronic kidney disease.

Below a GFR of 60, health complications from chronic kidney disease are much more likely to occur. The good news is that Stage 3 kidney disease is completely reversible. There is no reason why someone who is paying even the smallest amount of attention to their health, shouldn't be aware of the problem in time and be able to reverse it. We know that having even a mildly elevated protein level in the urine directly increases the risk for heart attack and stroke and premature death.[10] In fact, every decrease in kidney function directly relates to increased sickness and increased risk of death from all causes. But, again, the good news is that this condition is reversible.

> Many people today have health issues with their kidneys, but most of them are not aware of it. Why? Because there are often no obvious symptoms.

Many individuals whose kidney function is impaired by a third or a half have no symptoms. You can live pretty well with only one kidney, but not if that one kidney is functioning at only 50 percent efficiency as you age.

DIET AND KIDNEY DISEASE

One of the critical health challenges in the United States today is the fact that only 7 percent of the average American diet comes from whole, unprocessed foods such as fresh fruit and vegetables. It is amazing that the general population is as healthy as it is, because people are eating very little of the foods that were designed to heal the body and restore us to health. That is a major reason so many are developing problems with diabetes, hypertension, heart disease, and autoimmune disease. Dairy and animal products make up

42 percent of the average U.S. diet, and 51 percent comes from refined and processed foods.[11]

> For optimal health, we should be getting at least 80 percent of our calories from fruits, vegetables, beans, and whole grains, while limiting animal products as much as possible. In fact, the most healthful diet would not include animal products at all.

Those societies around the world who consume the least amount of animal protein—5 percent to 7 percent of total calories—are the healthiest societies. We should reduce our consumption of animal products at least to those amounts, if we don't eliminate them entirely.

Instead of making up 43 percent of our diet, refined and processed foods should be no more than 10 percent. These should be our dietary goals in order to optimize health and reduce our risk of such diseases as diabetes, hypertension, and heart disease. The above stats change from year to year, but unless we, as individuals, make a dramatic departure from the Standard American Diet (SAD), we are not going to be healthy.

STRATEGIES FOR REVERSING CHRONIC KIDNEY DISEASE

The reality is that 59 percent of Americans will suffer from kidney disease in their lifetime according to statistics published in May 2014.[12] Researchers at Johns Hopkins University have identified kidney disease as a huge problem and have warned that we are heading toward widespread chronic kidney disease unless we take definite steps to halt and reverse this process.

What can we do to meet this crisis?

A study published in 2014 in the *Clinical Journal of the American Society of Nephrology* looked at more than 6,000 patients who were in the final stages of chronic kidney disease.[13] The study found that walking dramatically lowered the risk of dying from the disease or requiring dialysis. Each incremental increase in walking during a given week dramatically increased the chances of doing well and being healthy, decreased the risk of dying during that year, and also decreased the possibility of having to go on dialysis.

> Walking one or two days per week lowered the risk of death during that year by 17 percent. Walking three to four times a week lowered the risk by 28 percent, and walking five to six times a week decreased the risk of premature death by 58 percent. A daily exercise program is critical to dealing with chronic kidney disease.

In spite of the well-known benefits of exercise, more than 80 percent of Americans are not exercising enough. Worse yet, less than 5 percent of adults are getting thirty minutes of exercise every day.[16] I know we are all busy, but exercise is vitally important and an easy thing to put into practice if we really want to optimize our health. I recently had a patient who is at significant risk for a heart attack or stroke. I asked him how much exercise he was getting.

"Well," he answered, "I mow the lawn."

He is retired. He stays active, and I commended him for that. Staying active is critical to health and longevity. Simply being up on our feet at least once every hour helps lower inflammation,[15] but in and of itself, that is clearly not enough exercise. We need to have a planned exercise program.

We must supplement our normal daily activity with at least thirty minutes of planned exercise. Without it, our body suffers. But even the fittest among us need to avoid sitting for extended periods. Even when exercising for thirty to sixty minutes daily, sitting for over an hour increases inflammatory levels in our body.

The bottom line is that "sitting is the new smoking," and we should plan to get up and move for at least two or three minutes after every hour of sitting. Better yet, get a standing desk, with a mini-stepper, and stay active throughout the day even when reading or on the computer!

Another factor is so critical for the kidneys that a continuing education course was developed around it. A report published on *Medscape* showed that chronic kidney disease starts to advance from Stage 3 into Stage 4 when this miracle nutrient drops.[16] I'm talking about Vitamin D. As we saw in Chapter 4, sunlight and Vitamin D kill bacteria, protect against pneumonia, and fight tuberculosis. In fact, Vitamin D has been shown to cure tuberculosis when added to the normal tuberculosis medications. It adds years to our life. It synchronizes hormones, beautifies our skin, prevents certain cancers and multiple sclerosis, fights binge eating, drives away depression, and prevents falls in the elderly. It protects our bones and lowers the risk of hip fractures, increases agility, makes the muscles stronger, builds the immune system, and helps prevent or even reverse chronic kidney disease. Yes, Vitamin D is like a wonder drug that provides all these amazing benefits. Yet it has been getting some bad press recently, creating confusion in many people's minds.

THE CALCIUM CALCIFICATION PARADOX

I continue to believe in the benefits of Vitamin D. My favorite definition of faith is holding on to something that you know to be true in spite of changing circumstances and moods.[17] The winds of change are always around us. We must be grounded in what we believe, and Vitamin D is an example of this.

One of the reasons Vitamin D is so critical to health is because of the calcium calcification paradox.[18] This refers to the fact that as we age, we develop osteoporosis at the very same time that calcium is hardening our arteries. Bone calcium loss leads to calcium buildup in the arteries and kidneys. How can that be?

During my professional training at Loma Linda University, we were all assigned to a cadaver in our anatomy class. My cadaver was that of a 45-year-old woman who had died of heart disease. We had to learn every organ, every part, of that cadaver inside and out. One particular day, my task was to dissect the heart and inspect the coronary arteries. As I did so, I noticed how hard the arteries were. Not having had much experience, I thought the arteries were hard just because they belonged to a cadaver.

The professor came to me and said, "Do you know what you're seeing? That's hardening of the arteries."

As I cut the artery along its length and opened it up, I found inside a hollow column of calcium with walls about one and a half millimeters thick. I was able to separate it right out of the artery. It was a thick, hardened, calcified tube. And I remember thinking, *If only this person had been made aware of her risk and been educated on how to reverse calcium and plaque buildup in her arteries!* Of course, conventional medical wisdom at the time held that it was impossible to reverse hardening of the arteries.

We had just had a lecture on how bones, which are essentially huge deposits of calcium in our bodies, can slowly disintegrate because of osteoporosis. I recall wondering, *Why can't we get rid of calcium in our arteries if the calcium in our bones can be depleted so easily?* It didn't make sense to me. Now we understand that there is this calcification paradox. When the Vitamin D in the blood gets low, the body's ability to draw calcium from our food or supplements, into the blood stream, is greatly diminished. And as the blood calcium starts to decrease, the body instantly reacts to avoid a low blood calcium level. Immediately the parathyroid gland releases its hormone, which travels to the bone and stimulates little cells, called osteoclasts, to chew up bone and spit it out into the blood.

That raises the calcium level. However, the extra calcium floating around in the blood increases the risk of hardening and calcifying the arteries and kidneys.

When Vitamin D levels are low, the parathyroid hormone is produced at a higher level. This draws calcium out of the bones promoting osteoporosis, and that extra calcium can end up in the artery walls and in the kidneys.

This is a major risk factor for the progression of chronic kidney disease. By optimizing Vitamin D in your system you can reverse this whole process and protect the arteries and kidneys.

If you eat plenty of green, leafy vegetables so that you are getting plenty of Vitamin K, you can further help the arteries get rid of calcium. If Vitamin K is at optimal levels, there is a Matrix Gla-Protein in the blood vessel walls that is able to inhibit calcification, get rid of calcium deposits, and begin changing that hard artery into a flexible, healthy, biologically younger artery.[19, 20] So we have to pay attention to the calcium calcification paradox. Don't make the mistake of thinking that you are not at risk for this. In fact, most adults aged 60 or older already have progressively enlarging deposits of calcium in their major arteries.[21] Inadequate levels of these nutrients strongly promote unhealthy calcification and many serious health problems, leading to premature disability and death from hypertension, congestive heart failure, and compromised blood flow to every part of the body including the brain, heart, spinal column, legs, sexual organs, and kidneys.[22, 23]

CHARCOAL AND KIDNEY DISEASE

There is another powerful, natural strategy available in dealing with chronic kidney disease and its complications. Believe it or not, it's charcoal. In Chapter 5 we discussed the power of charcoal in helping to detoxify the body and support healthy digestion. When I talk about the health benefits of charcoal, I sometimes get strange looks, because people think I'm talking about barbecue charcoal briquettes that are loaded with toxic-smelling chemical additives! No, I'm talking about medical-grade, activated charcoal that is used by hospital emergency departments as the universal anti-toxin and also for drug overdose cases.

In 2010, kidney doctors from all over the world attended the annual meeting of the American Society of Nephrology in San Diego, California.[24] The one presentation that got my attention that year was given by Dr. Valentina Kon, a pediatric kidney specialist and professor at Vanderbilt University. She presented her study showing that mice with damaged kidneys, and thus unable to fully detoxify the blood, quickly developed atherosclerosis and serious heart disease. But when powdered, activated charcoal was added to the diets of these mice, they didn't develop nearly as much heart disease even though they had compromised kidneys.[25] It was an interesting finding, because once chronic kidney disease reaches Stage 4, and especially Stage 5, there is little currently available in conventional medical practice to effectively treat and prevent the rapid progression of heart disease.[26] Another study also found that adding charcoal to the mice's diet greatly limited progression of their heart disease even when the treatment was delayed.[27] What was the significant factor producing these results?

The researchers found that after charcoal was added to the diet, the mice's cholesterol was still the same; the blood pressure was still the same. What changed dramatically was inflammation.

Charcoal treatment actually turned down the expression of genes that promoted inflammation.[28] For the most part, it is toxins in the blood that create inflammation.

The top lipidologists and research cardiologists understand that for plaque to begin to build up in the artery wall, there must first be toxins present.[29] The plaque is the result of white blood cells trying to remove toxins from the artery wall. As these white blood cells fill up with oxidized cholesterol and other toxic substances, they form into foam cells, causing plaque. These studies suggest a potential remedy that people can use to improve health in general, including all stages of chronic kidney disease. We need to address what is causing the toxicity.

I personally take what I call my "black shake" about once a week as a form of natural detoxification support. I take a heaping teaspoon of powdered activated charcoal and mix it thoroughly with about four ounces of cold water. It might look nasty, but it doesn't taste that bad.

More important, it's one more thing that gives me confidence that I'm supporting my body's need to eliminate toxins and inflammatory chemicals. Of course, if my blood tests showed high levels of inflammation, or if I were at risk of heart disease, and especially if I had kidney disease, I would drink my "black shake" more often. A good time to take charcoal is at bedtime, but since charcoal can bind and de-activate medications as well as toxins, it should be used at least one hour after, or three hours before, taking any prescription medications.

THE IMPORTANCE OF LIFESTYLE CHANGES

At a small medical conference a visiting nephrologist was giving a talk to our group about a new blood pressure medication. Looking at us, he asked, "What is the average number of blood pressure medications needed to properly treat hypertension?"

After a moment, he continued by saying, "We all need to stop telling our patients that they can resolve their blood pressure problem with one medication, because that rarely happens. We need to stop telling our patients that they can control their blood pressure problems with even two medications." He went on to say that in nephrology and the treatment of hypertension, it often takes three or four different types of blood pressure medications to control blood pressure—unless, he added, the patient gets "religion" in the form of lifestyle medicine.

I was surprised when he said that. He had jokingly made fun of lifestyle medicine, yet he had admitted that it is the only alternative to using multiple medications! He had unintentionally underlined the most important factor in treating hypertension which is one of the main causes of heart disease, strokes, and kidney failure.

Just like in diabetes, heart disease, and cholesterol management, the first-line therapy—the treatment that is officially established as the first step in treatment—is lifestyle medicine. But far too many doctors have little faith that their patients will make the necessary lifestyle changes, and therefore they don't even try to comply with the therapy guidelines.

In dealing with blood pressure, it is important not to over medicate. As I have worked with many patients over the last twenty-five years who have gone through intensive lifestyle medicine programs, I have noticed that initially patients who are on blood pressure medications are often doing well and feeling great. Then after about six weeks of following a comprehensive wellness program, they will often say, "I just don't feel good anymore. Something is wrong."

This is what often happens. They have made such dramatic health improvements to their circulatory system that now even decreased levels of blood pressure medication have the potential to drop their blood pressure too low. Now, these medications are actually placing them at risk. Don't misunderstand.

I am not saying that patients should never be on blood pressure medication. I am saying that once a person has addressed the cause of the problem, they need to work with their primary care physician to adjust their medication or they will likely become over medicated.

Over medication can make them feel so bad that they don't want to follow the wellness program anymore. And if they discontinue the lifestyle changes, they will go right back to needing the medications.

DIET MAKES A DIFFERENCE

Dr. Neil Barnard is director of the Physician's Committee for Responsible Medicine and is a professor at Georgetown University. He received a grant to work with a group of diabetics to determine the best diet for reversing diabetes and helping to optimize blood sugars. During a three-month controlled intervention trial,he compared the American Diabetes Association (ADA) diet with what he referred to as "the best diet." Diabetic patients, with their spouses, were randomly assigned to two groups and met two evenings every week for three months at which they had catered meals. One group received meals based on the ADA recommended diet. The other group ate Dr. Barnard's "best diet." The main difference between the two diets was that the ADA diet included thirty grams of fiber and 200 mg of cholesterol from chicken or fish, whereas the "best diet" included no cholesterol and sixty to seventy grams of fiber. The "best diet" was 100 percent plant based.

The group on the American Diabetic Association diet improved in several important areas. Blood sugars got better without any changes in medications and they lost an average of 8-½ pounds. However, their kidney function, the amount of protein that leaked from the kidneys into the urine, got worse even after better blood sugar control and weight loss.

In spite of the fact that they ended up needing much less diabetes medication, the 100 percent plant-based diet group had a 59 percent greater improvement in their blood sugars than did the ADA diet group which had no change in medication. They also lost an average of sixteen pounds, almost double the weight loss of the ADA-diet group. Kidney function for this group improved; they had less protein in their urine.

All these changes took place in three months. So the diet that we consume very quickly influences kidney function in a powerful way.

We cannot have good health unless we have healthy kidneys. And unless we have healthy kidneys, we cannot properly remove the toxins that our bodies are constantly exposed to.

In order to have healthy kidneys, we have to have healthy circulation. But we cannot have good circulation with inflammation and toxins causing damage to our blood vessels, immune system, and kidneys. We will learn more about how toxins influence auto-immune disease in Chapter 9 and how to support the liver's role of detoxification in Chapter 10.

Fiber was one of the important variables between the diets in Dr. Barnard's study. A key wellness goal is to optimize fiber, especially since it binds toxic substances and speeds the removal of waste products from the body. I recommend that my patients get forty to fifty grams of fiber from whole foods daily. If you regularly use beans, peas, or lentils in your diet, you are going to be getting eight grams of fiber for every one-half cup serving. If you don't use beans in your diet very often, you are not going to get a lot of fiber.

You can also get fiber in vegetables; one cup of non-starchy vegetables provides about two grams of fiber. One-half cup of grains will give your three grams of fiber, as will a half cup of fruit or a medium apple.

When you eat a meal, do the math. Try to get at least ten grams of fiber for breakfast and fifteen grams of fiber for lunch and also for dinner. These are minimums.

Fiber is what helps clean out your system and further protect your kidneys and circulation. Getting the right amount of whole-food fiber is a key to an effective wellness program, so make sure you are getting enough fiber in your daily diet.

IS REVERSAL POSSIBLE?

In 2004 the president of a large regional medical society invited me to speak at its upcoming conference. There would be 500 physicians and health professionals in attendance from all around the Pacific Rim. He asked me to speak about reversing diabetes through nutrition. Now, I knew that this was a controversial subject—at least it was at that time. I knew the potential political consequences of speaking on this topic. "Are you sure you want me to talk about that?" I asked.

"Oh, yes," he replied. "They'll love it."

So I agreed. When I walked into the hall to give my presentation, an internationally known geneticist and researcher had just finished speaking. Now it was my turn. I gave what I thought was a good ninety-minute overview of how nutrition can actually reverse diabetes. During my presentation, I showed a short clip from the documentary, *Supersize Me*.[30] If you haven't seen it, you should.

The producer of the documentary decided to eat nothing but food from McDonald's for thirty days. It almost killed him, literally. He gained twenty-nine pounds in thirty days; his liver enzymes went through the roof. He had three doctors checking on him separately, none of the three knew about the other two. Each doctor told him, "You're ruining your liver. Whatever you're doing, stop doing it." One asked him, "Are you drinking vodka all night?" It's an interesting documentary. In the film, the producer interviews two bariatric surgeons who state that the only known procedure in medicine that can cure diabetes is gastric bypass surgery.

In my talk, I clarified that I was not recommending bariatric surgery for diabetes treatment. Rather, I was countering the conventional medical wisdom that diabetes could not be reversed. While I believe that lifestyle strategies like nutrition and exercise are the optimal way to reverse diabetes, showing that interview, with the surgeons talking about their research, helped me demonstrate that a cure was very much possible.

At the end of my presentation, the chairman of the scientific panel for that session came to the podium. I assumed he was going to take questions for me from the audience. But he had something to say first. "I want to clarify something," he said. "I completely disagree with Dr. Youngberg's presentation this afternoon."

You could have heard a pin drop! All 500 people in the audience were looking at me. They were looking at him. I was looking at him. He went on to explain himself. He wasn't upset with me or trying to make me look bad. He was just establishing what he believed. And, of course, that is what such conferences are all about—stating what you believe, what you think is accurate based on the scientific evidence.

While he was explaining his position, I was praying, "Lord, help me to know what to say. Help me know how to address this challenge and not take it personally."

The chairman acknowledged that the previous speaker, the internationally recognized geneticist, had stated in his talk that he believed we would, in the future, be able to reverse diabetes through the application of genetic engineering principles. As soon as I heard that, I knew exactly what I needed to say.

When he finished explaining why he disagreed with my presentation, I said, "Doctor, I appreciate your perspective." This man was a nephrologist, a kidney specialist. He had a renal dialysis unit right across the hall from our lifestyle medicine clinic. I saw him all the time. Knowing this, I understood why he would say that he didn't believe that diabetes was reversible.

You see, he was working daily with patients at the end of their experience with diabetes or hypertension. They were in the advanced stages of the disease. He had never seen diabetes reversed in his patients. On the other hand, my goal in working with diabetic patients was to reverse the disease, not merely manage symptoms.

As a result, I had seen diabetes reversed in many, many patients. Our perspectives were entirely different because we dealt with opposite ends of the spectrum of the disease.

We were like two blind men in a room with an elephant trying to describe it, when we were having completely different experiences with that "elephant."

So in reply, I said to him, "Doctor, I believe it is critical that we not destroy hope in our patients. If we tell our patients, "You are probably are not going to make it. We'll do everything we can to help you, but all we have is more insulin, more blood pressure medications, more cholesterol-lowering medicines," what effect is that going to have on the patient? He or she is probably going to go home depressed, hopeless, and continue to eat unhealthfully, avoid exercise, and do none of the things they need to do to become healthy again. We cannot destroy hope in our patients."

Then I added, "I'm glad that we have had an internationally recognized geneticist talk about the potential of genetic engineering in reversing diabetes, because that is exactly how nutritional and lifestyle medicine works.

It reengineers genetic risk by changing the way genes function." Fortunately, the chairman chose not to respond further to my comments, and we moved on to taking question from the audience.

Two days after this conference, I was driving to work, listening to the morning news. To my amazement, there was a news item of a major study reported in the *Journal of the American Medical Association,* showing that 77 percent of diabetics who had undergone gastric bypass surgery had completely resolved their diabetes. Among those with high blood pressure, 62 percent had resolved the problem. High cholesterol was improved in 70 percent, and 86 percent had taken care of their sleep apnea.[31]

I started thinking about how I could get this information to the nephrologist who worked next door and who had disagreed with me at the medical conference earlier. I parked my car, went inside, and got on the elevator. There was one person already on the elevator—the nephrologist!

My initial impulse was to rub it in. "Hey, did you see the new *JAMA* article that just came out?" But I thought better of it. I knew he would see the article soon enough. And he did. Within a month, he and I were collaborating on diabetes research.

GOOD HEALTH DEPENDS ON YOU

It's exciting to me how much we have learned about diabetes and kidney disease in the last ten years. We have learned that our potential to reverse disease is great. Our potential to prevent problems is even greater. If we are willing to pay attention to our bodies and the principles of health, we can do amazing things. We need to enjoy each day in a way that gives us even more joy tomorrow. That is what health and wellness is all about. It's not about "Oh, I can't eat that!" or "Oh, I have to go exercise again!"

Health and wellness isn't a matter of the things we can't do or the things we have to do. It's about experiencing optimal joy. It's about enjoying a level of health and wellness that allows us to live life to the fullest. We can't have that kind of full, rich life unless we have optimal health.

Experiencing good health is learning how to make choices that will bring you lasting happiness and joy. In the end, only *you* can do that; no one else can do it for you.

CHAPTER SUMMARY

>> When facing health problems, it's important to focus on root causes rather than on superficial symptoms.

>> Four important tests for kidney disease are the Glomerular Filtration Rate (GFR), the Blood Urea Nitrogen test (BUN), the Creatinine test, and the Microalbumin Urine test.

>> At some point in their life, more than half of Americans will suffer from kidney disease, but you don't have to be one of them.

>> Even in patients in the final stages of chronic kidney disease, walking dramatically lowers the risk of dying from the disease or requiring dialysis. Walking five to six times a week decreases the risk by 58 percent.

>> Less than 5 percent of adults are getting thirty minutes of exercise every day. You can be one of those 5 percent. It's only thirty minutes, and anyone can do it!

>> Chronic bone calcium loss leads to osteoporosis, but also simultaneously leads to calcium buildup in the arteries and kidneys. This is known as the calcium paradox.

>> Optimizing Vitamin D intake can greatly slow bone calcium loss and stop progression of chronic kidney disease.

>> A 100 percent plant-based diet, providing high levels of many nutrients and whole-food fiber, is shown to help reverse chronic kidney disease.

>> Foods rich in Vitamin K activate GLA protein matrix in blood vessel walls that prevents and reverses calcium deposits in artery walls and kidneys.

>> Lab tests that measure inflammation in the blood predict risk for progression of chronic kidney disease.

>> Untreated dental problems such as gingivitis and periodontal disease are significant sources of inflammation and toxicity for the entire body, and especially increase the risk of strokes, heart attacks, and kidney disease.

>> Activated, powdered charcoal is effective at binding toxins that cause inflammation, thus greatly minimizing the risk of atherosclerosis caused by kidney disease.

>> Charcoal taken orally helps turn off genes that promote inflammation.

>> Being aware of our risk factors and making good choices help us enjoy a level of health and wellness that allows us to live life to the fullest.

ENDNOTES

1 Cowie, C, et al, "Full Accounting of Diabetes and Pre-Diabetes in the U.S. Population in 1988-1994 and 2005-2006," *Diabetes Care,* 32 (2009) 287–294.

2 Castelli, W, "The new pathophysiology of coronary artery disease", *Am J Cardiology,* November 26, 1998 Volume 82, Issue 10, Supplement 2, Pages 60–65.

3 Stratton, Irene, et al, "Association of Glycaemia with Macrovascular and Microvascular Complications of Type 2 Diabetes (UKPDS 35): Prospective Observational Study," *BMJ,* 321.7258 (2000): 405-412.

4 El-Shinnawi, U, "Associations between periodontitis and systemic inflammatory diseases: response to treatment", Recent Pat Endocr Metab Immune Drug Discov. 2013 Sep;7(3):169-88.

5 Gener, I, "Periodontal Disease: A Covert Source of Inflammation in Chronic Kidney Disease Patients," *International Journal of Nephrology,* vol. 2013, Article ID 515796, 6 pages, 2013. doi:10.1155/2013/515796

6 Friedewald, V, "The American Journal of Cardiology and Journal of Periodontology Editors' Consensus: periodontitis and atherosclerotic cardiovascular disease", J Periodontol. 2009;80:1021–1032.

7 Pingping, L, "LTB4 promotes insulin resistance in obese mice by acting on macrophages, hepatocytes and myocytes", *Nature Medicine* (2015) doi:10.1038/nm.3800 Published online 23 February 2015

8 Colotta, C, "Cancer-related inflammation, the seventh hallmark of cancer: links to genetic instability", Carcinogenesis (2009) 30 (7): 1073-1081 first published online May 25, 2009 doi:10.1093/carcin/bgp127

9 Levey, A, "National Kidney Foundation Practice Guidelines for Chronic Kidney Disease: Evaluation, Classification, and Stratification", *Ann Intern Med.* 2003;139(2):137-147. doi:10.7326/0003-4819-139-2-200307150-00013

10 Gemma Currie, "Proteinuria and its relation to cardiovascular disease", *Int J Nephrol Renovasc Dis.* 2014; 7: 13–24. Published online 2013 Dec 21. doi: 10.2147/IJNRD.S40522PMCID: PMC3873205

11 Joel Fuhrman, *Eat to Live: The Revolutionary Formula for Fast and Sustained Weight Loss* (Boston: Little, Brown, 2003).

12 Morgan E. Grams, "Lifetime Incidence of CKD Stages 3-5 in the United States", *Am J Kidney Dis.* 2013;62(2):245-252.

13 I-Ru Chen "Association of Walking with Survival and Renal Replacement Therapy among Patients with CKD Stages 3-5", CJASN July 07, 2014 9): (7) 1183-1189; published ahead of print May 15, 2014, doi:10.2215/CJN.09810913

14 Troiano, R, "Physical activity in the United States measured by accelerometer", *Med Sci Sports Exerc* 2008;40:181–188.

15 Yates T et al. Self-reported sitting time and markers of inflammation, insulin resistance, and adiposity. *Am J Prev Med.* 2012 Jan;42(1):1-7.

16 Bryan R. Kestenbaum, "Chronic Kidney Disease Expert Column: Vitamin D Metabolism and Treatment in Chronic Kidney Disease", *Medscape Nephrology.* 2008; Posted 03/25/2008 http://www.medscape.com/viewarticle/571558

17 Paraphrased from C. S. Lewis, *Mere Christianity*, pg. 126.

18 Persy, V, "Vascular calcification and bone disease: the calcification paradox",*Trends Mol Med.* 2009 Sep;15(9):405-16. doi: 10.1016/j.molmed.2009.07.001. Epub 2009 Sep 3.

19 Schurgers, L, "Vitamin K-dependent carboxylation of matrix Gla-protein: a crucial switch to control ectopic mineralization", *Trends in Molecular Medicine*, Volume 19 , Issue 4 , 217 – 226, April 2013.

20 Theuwissen, E, "Thematic Review Series: Vitamin K: The Role of Vitamin K in Soft-Tissue Calcification", *Adv Nutr* March 2012 Vol. 3, 166-173; doi:10.3945/an.111.001628

21 Allison, M, "Patterns and risk factors for systemic calcified atherosclerosis", *Arterioscler Thromb Vasc Biol.* 2004; 24: 331–336.

22 Wayhs R, "High coronary artery calcium scores pose an extremely elevated risk for hard events", J Am Coll Cardiol. 2002; 39: 225–230.

23 Demer, L, "Basic Science for Clinicians: Vascular Calcification: Pathobiology of a Multifaceted Disease", *Circulation.* 2008;117:2938-2948, doi:10.1161/CIRCULATIONAHA.107.743161

24 2010 at the American Society of Nephrology's 42nd Annual Meeting and Scientific Exposition in San Diego, CA.

25 Yamarnoto, S, "Oral activated charcoal adsorbent (AST-120) ameliorates extent and instability of atherosclerosis accelerated by kidney disease in apolipoprotein E-deficient mice", Nephrol Dial Transplant (2011) 0: 1–7 doi: 10.1093/ndt/gfq759

26 Fellstrom B, et al. "Rosuvastatin and cardiovascular events in patients undergoing hemodialysis", N Engl J Med 2009; 360: 1395–1407.

27 Fujii, H, "Oral charcoal adsorbent (AST-120) prevents progression of cardiac damage in chronic kidney disease through suppression of oxidative stress", Nephrol. Dial. Transplant. (2009) 24 (7): 2089-2095 first published online February 2, 2009 doi:10.1093/ndt/gfp007

28 Yamamoto, S, "Oral activated charcoal adsorbent (AST-120) ameliorates extent and instability of atherosclerosis accelerated by kidney disease in apolipoprotein E-deficient mice", *Nephrol Dial Transplant* (2011) 0: 1–7 doi: 10.1093/ndt/gfq759

29 "Optimizing Patient Cardiovascular Care with the Hunter Heart Profile," a 2014 presentation by Paul Ziajka, M.D., Ph.D., Director of The Florida Lipid Institute; Diplomat of the American Board of Clinical Lipidology; President of the South East Lipid Association.

30 "Supersize Me," directed by Morgan Spurlock (United States: Samuel Goldwyn Films, 2004), DVD.

31 Buchwald, Henry, et al, "Bariatric Surgery: A Systematic Review and Meta-analysis," *The Journal of the American Medical Association*, 292.14 (2004): 1724-1737.

NINE

Friendly Fire

THE AUTOIMMUNE EPIDEMIC

JIM CAME TO SEE ME ABOUT FOUR YEARS AGO. He didn't have any real complaints; he just wanted to check out his overall health and see if there were any concerns he wasn't aware of. We did some comprehensive lab tests, and the results that came back upset Jim. He had early diabetes; there was no question about it. But he didn't have any symptoms that he could feel. So he decided to ignore it. He chose to continue his current lifestyle and just forget about it.

A few months ago, however, Jim started experiencing some symptoms. He was losing weight even though he'd always had to struggle a little to keep his weight down. Now he was eating more, but losing weight. He thought that was kind of odd. He noticed frequent urination. His energy was low; he just didn't feel good. He started thinking about the tests we had run some four years earlier and decided that maybe it was time to check things again. He came in, and we discovered that now Jim had out-of-control diabetes with blood sugars in the 300 to 400 range!

REVERSING THE IRREVERSIBLE

There is a test I believe everyone should have. *Everyone.* It has a scientific, academic name—the hemoglobin A1C test. But I call it the sticky sugar test or the sugar glazed protein test. It measures how much blood sugar irreversibly binds and literally glazes to the hemoglobin proteins found within the red blood cells. This glazing that occurs, even with minimal spikes in blood sugar, is referred to as glycosylation or glycation. The AIC test is typically used to determine how well diabetics have controlled their blood sugars over the last three to four months. But the A1C test also helps us to estimate how much sugar is binding to proteins and fats everywhere blood flows throughout our body,[1] and that is why anyone—not just diabetics—can benefit from this test. The A1C is an easily measured form of Advanced Glycated Endproducts (AGEs) that are produced by sugar glazing to proteins. This glazing stimulates oxidation, inflammation and other toxic reactions that promote free radical damage to hormones and many other proteins throughout the body.[2] AGEs also accelerate aging, in part by the glazing of sugar to LDL cholesterol,[3] strongly promoting plaque buildup and cardiovascular disease. This process is also known to initiate and aggravate autoimmune disease,[4] including autoimmune destruction of beta cells in the pancreas, thus limiting the ability to produce insulin.[5]

Excess sugar also glazes to the proteins in our cell membranes.[6] It's the proteins in the cell membranes, the outer walls of our cells, that determine the function and the inter-relationship between all cells.[7]

Keeping our proteins healthy is critical. It's the individual proteins in our blood and tissues that collectively determine how well our body functions. In fact, we can say that protein is equivalent to life. It's literally a life and death matter.

But when sugar irreversibly binds to proteins anywhere in the body, it changes the way the protein works. Proteins are like little machines, and machines work differently based on how they're designed, how the parts are configured. If sugar sticks to proteins, it permanently twists their configuration, and they no longer work the way they are supposed to. This sticky sugar test measures how sugar in the blood is binding to hemoglobin, one of the most prevalent proteins in the bloodstream. Hemoglobin is the protein that incorporates the mineral iron at its core and therefore attracts oxygen into the red blood cells so that they can carry that life-giving oxygen to every cell within our body.

Sugar in the blood is constantly, and in a limited way, binding with proteins in and on our cells. But when blood sugar levels are higher than normal, excessive amounts of this irreversible binding take place. When are the blood sugars most likely to run high? Right after meals. Within thirty to sixty minutes after beginning your meal, your blood sugar is typically going to be at its peak, and that provides an opportunity to gradually reverse the irreversible binding of sugars to proteins.

How can that be? If it's "irreversible," how can we reverse it? How can we reverse diabetes, plaque buildup, and autoimmune problems if glycosylation, this glazing effect of sugar to proteins, is indeed irreversible?

The answer is simple. Our bodies were made to constantly recreate themselves. That's an important concept to grasp. Eventually those cells that have been irreversibly bound by excess sugar will go through their lifecycle. For red blood cells, the lifecycle is about 120 days. After an average of 120 days, those red blood cells will die, break apart, and the body will make new ones. That's why all of us have the opportunity to be recreated. Our bodies are always recreating themselves. So if we give the body what it needs, it can actually reverse the irreversible.

A1C and AGE levels become elevated with high blood sugars. But did you know that we can get unhealthful levels of AGEs directly from the foods we eat? Yes, one reason foods are unhealthful for us is the amount of preformed AGEs they contain even before we eat them.

So what can we do?

First, avoid highly processed carbohydrate-rich foods, especially those containing excess refined sugars. Second, avoid or highly limit animal products. Animal-derived foods that are high in fat and protein are generally AGE-rich and prone to excess AGE formation during cooking. In contrast, vegetables and fruits contain relatively few AGEs even after cooking. AGEs formed from high blood sugars or from the foods we eat represent pathogenic compounds that are linked to the initiation and progression of many chronic diseases.[8]

TRANSFORMATION IN THREE MONTHS

An optimal hemoglobin A1C for an individual who does not have diabetes should measure 5 percent or a little less.[9, 10] Studies show that the risk of cardiovascular disease starts to creep up as glycosylation in the form of hemoglobin A1C goes above 4.6 percent even in those without diabetes or prediabetes.[11] However, the official diagnosis of prediabetes begins at an A1C of 5.7 percent.

> Remember, at least half of individuals between the ages of 40 and 59 already have prediabetes, as do two-thirds of those 60 to 74 years of age, and three-fourths of those over 75 years old.[12] Yet the vast majority of them are unaware of their problem.

Unfortunately, these statistics represent the new "normal." That is what we expect to find in those age groups. So ideally we want the hemoglobin A1C test, the sticky sugar test, to be 5 percent or less.

When we did the second round of testing on Jim, some years after his initial tests, we found his hemoglobin A1C level was 12.1 percent. He knew that the optimal level is 5 percent and that a diagnosis of diabetes begins at 6.5 percent. He also knew that every percentage point above 5 means an increase in the blood glucose level of thirty-plus points. A normal hemoglobin A1C reading of 5 percent represents a blood glucose level of 80. At 6 percent, you're right in the middle of prediabetes, on your way to diabetes, which begins at 6.5 percent, and that means your average fasting blood sugar is about 126. If you're at a 7 percent hemoglobin A1C, your average blood sugar is 150. Jim's hemoglobin A1C level was 12.1 percent. That meant that his average blood sugars were at least 300. In reality, Jim's fasting blood sugars were actually running somewhere between 350 and 400 on a regular basis.

Every percentage point above a normal hemoglobin A1C of 5 percent increases the risk of nerve damage by 37 percent. This nerve damage leads to neuropathy, nerve pain, and possible amputations. The risk factors for vision loss and kidney disease also increase by 37 percent for each percentage point increase in the hemoglobin A1C level. The risk for heart attacks increases by

14 percent, and the risk for all diabetes-related deaths increases 21 percent.[13]

Jim was looking at his hemoglobin A1C of 12.1 percent, knowing that his risk of premature death due to diabetes had just gone up more than 120 percent. Now he became motivated. Now he recognized how foolish it had been to ignore the warning signs four years earlier. Jim began making significant changes in his lifestyle. Knowing that after-meal blood sugar spikes have the largest influence on the A1C level, and more broadly on AGE sugar glazing of body proteins,[14] Jim started exercising thirty minutes after each meal. He completely changed his diet and started eating primarily whole, unprocessed plant foods. He was going all out.

Jim knew he had to "pull out all the stops" to be successful. No amount of "baby steps" was going to get Jim where he wanted to be. Healthful, well-balanced meals are less likely to spike blood sugars, and they are also low in preformed AGEs. Incredibly, processed foods and animal products are a major source of dietary AGEs, especially when exposed to extended high heat and low moisture. Alternatively, brief heating times, low temperatures, high moisture, and/or pre-exposure to an acidified environment like lemon juice are great ways to limit AGE formation in food. A significant reduction of dietary AGEs can be achieved by eating more legumes, vegetables, fruits, and whole grains—and by avoiding solid fats, fatty meats, and highly processed foods.[15]

In only three months, Jim brought his hemoglobin A1C down to 6 percent! A dramatic reversal!

By the way, it takes more than three months to clear out all those old cells that have been irreversibly bound by high sugar levels and damaged by unhealthful foods.

So in another month, Jim's hemoglobin A1C would be even lower. By that standard, Jim had essentially reversed his diabetes.

Of course, that doesn't mean that Jim could now stop following his new lifestyle changes and go back to his old way of living. What would happen if he did that? His diabetes would go right back to that irreversible condition.

As Jim's story tells us, the good news is that even when we're stubborn and resistant to change, the irreversible can still be reversed—if we act in time.

GOOD NEWS OR BAD NEWS?

With all the changes taking place in his life, Jim was excited and eager to optimize every area of his health. We decided to do some genetic testing for advanced risk markers related to cardiovascular disease and take advantage of the cutting edge science and tests that are available today. When we did, we discovered that Jim had a significant mutation to the Apolipoprotein E gene (Apo E). Having the Apo E4 mutation instead of the normal Apo E3 non-mutated gene, doubles the risk of cardiovascular disease and exponentially increases the risk of Alzheimer's disease. The normal, healthy Apo E3 gene codes for the production of protein molecules that help break down and remove the beta amyloid plaques that are toxic to brain cells and that are associated with Alzheimer's disease.[16]

I told Jim that each of us has one copy of the Apo E gene from each parent. If one parent gives us a normal copy of Apo E and our other parent gives us the mutated copy of Apo E, we end up with an Apo E3/E4 combination. This combination statistically increases our risk of Alzheimer's an average of two to four times.

If both parents give us a mutated copy, we end up with Apo E4/E4 which is associated with a dramatically increased risk—from five to thirty-four times greater![17]

I carefully explained to Jim that he had two copies (E4/E4) of the mutated gene. Statistically Jim had up to a 3,000 percent increased risk of Alzheimer's disease!

At first glance, this was terrible news. But I said, "You know, Jim, this can be good news!"

He had developed a trusting relationship with me by this time. I had told him that dramatic transformation could take place in his health if he focused on lifestyle intervention. He had seen that happen just as I had promised. His physical symptoms had improved tremendously. He was thinner and healthier. He trusted me, but he was puzzled how I could consider it to be good news that his risk of Alzheimer's was greatly increased. Like most people would, Jim reasoned, *After all I've done to improve my health, I get thrown this curve ball of a substantially increased risk of Alzheimer's.*

But that perception isn't totally accurate. The increased risk of Alzheimer's was true, *only if nothing had changed in Jim's approach to his health. Only if Jim hadn't already been doing all those things that had dramatically transformed his health.*

I told Jim that he was not alone. About one in four Americans has at least one copy of the Apo E mutation.[18] It was important for Jim to understand that at least 20 percent of those who have this Apo E4 mutation do *not* develop Alzheimer's and also that many individuals develop Alzheimer's even though they do not carry this gene mutation. The key was to recognize and identify the actual lifestyle triggers that would powerfully silence his disease-causing genes and to more effectively activate his health promoting genes.

Jim came to understand that all the lifestyle changes he had been making had not only significantly helped him reverse his diabetes, but even more importantly it would be helping him prevent serious cardiovascular disease and the potential risk of developing Alzheimer's.

If he hadn't taken the initiative to address the underlying causes of his diabetes, he would have never learned about this genetic mutation that he had carried since birth. He wouldn't have thought about what he should be doing to deal with it.

A gene is not what primarily determines our risk; it's what we do with that gene. It's the choices we make that relate to that gene. It's our environment and the nutritional and attitudinal exposures around that gene that determine whether that gene is turned on or turned off.

If you had the opportunity to find out whether you had a major gene for Alzheimer's or some other disease, would you want to know? I believe it is in our best interest to know. I would want to know as soon as possible so that I could start trying to find solutions that could dramatically alter my risk of future disease. See Chapter 12 for more information on Apo E and gene testing.

DETOXIFICATION AND ALZHEIMER'S DISEASE

The tests Jim took, these advanced biomarkers for cardiac risk, are basically indicators of inflammation. Numerous studies show that the markers of inflammation represent triggers for cardiovascular disease, which is the number one cause of death in the world. Heart disease is driven by inflammation. Inflammation, as we've seen in previous chapters, is a common factor in most chronic and acute disease.

Not only is it a critical marker for disease, but the presence of inflammation in the body tells us that we need to find the cause. The risk for Alzheimer's is very strongly related to inflammation.[19] An impaired capacity to eliminate toxins or toxic compounds[20] and a lack of nutritional factors[21, 22, 23] are key promoters of Alzheimer's. These are also factors that promote heart disease.

Chapter 10 will be dealing with detoxification. If you read the medical literature today, you will quickly discover that if your body is not effective in going through its detoxification process, day in and day out, hourly, minute-by-minute, your risk for just about every illness goes up dramatically.

> We're beginning to understand that one of the drivers of cardiovascular disease and autoimmune conditions is the inability of the body to get rid of normal, everyday toxins and to get nutrients to the cells appropriately.

That's why all the things we've been discussing—digestion, circulation, kidney function, nutrition, etc.—are critical in dealing not only with heart disease, but also with autoimmunity. In fact, we're learning now that Alzheimer's is actually an autoimmune process as well.[24] The more we learn, the more we find that all the body's processes come together; they all affect each other.

Research has shown that Alzheimer's disease can actually be caused and triggered by the common Herpes Simplex Virus Type 1,[25, 26] a mild infection that is found in 54 percent of Americans.[27]

That's why, as a population, we need to think long and hard about our exposure to these viruses and rethink what is acceptable in terms of sexual practices. Historically, HSV-1 was also called oral herpes, an infection in the mouth, and HSV-2 was called genital herpes. In a study done on U.S. college students, the percentage of genital herpes cases attributable to HSV-1 increased from 31 percent in 1993 to 78 percent in 2001.[28] In another study, nearly 60 percent of genital herpes infections were caused by HSV-1.[29]

How we relate to each other dramatically increases our risk of various forms of what are considered mild, inconsequential viral infections that are strongly implicated in the slow, gradual development of Alzheimer's disease and other autoimmune-related conditions. This is especially true if we have certain genotypes. That's why I strongly encourage everyone to take advantage of genetic testing.

If we have the Apo E4 mutation on the Apo lipoprotein gene, it means we need to more carefully evaluate our risk of low-grade infections and do everything possible to subdue them.[30]

THE AUTOIMMUNE EPIDEMIC

An autoimmune disorder occurs when the body's immune system attacks and destroys healthy body tissue by mistake. When you have an autoimmune disorder, your immune system does not distinguish between healthy tissue and the harmful antigens found in bacteria, viruses, toxins, cancer cells, and foreign tissues.[31]

As a result, the body sets off a reaction that destroys normal tissues. There are more than eighty types of autoimmune disorders that can affect essentially every system, organ, and tissue in our body.

TABLE OF COMMON AUTOIMMUNE DISEASES[32]

The following are some of the more common autoimmune diseases:

>> **RHEUMATOID ARTHRITIS**—inflammation of joints and surrounding tissues.

>> **SYSTEMIC LUPUS ERYTHEMATOSUS**—affects skin, joints, kidneys, brain, and other organs.

>> **MULTIPLE SCLEROSIS**—affects the brain and spinal cord.

>> **CELIAC SPRUE DISEASE**—a reaction to gluten (found in wheat, rye, and barley) that causes damage to the lining of the small intestine.

>> **PERNICIOUS ANEMIA**—a decrease in red blood cells caused by the inability to absorb vitamin B12.

>> **VITILIGO**—white patches on the skin caused by loss of pigment.

>> **SCLERODERMA**—a connective tissue disease that causes changes in skin, blood vessels, muscles, and internal organs.

>> **PSORIASIS**—a skin condition that causes redness and irritation as well as thick, flaky, silver-white patches.

>> **INFLAMMATORY BOWEL DISEASE**—a group of inflammatory diseases of the colon and small intestine.

>> **HASHIMOTO'S DISEASE**—inflammation of the thyroid gland.

>> **ADDISON'S DISEASE**—adrenal hormone insufficiency.

>> **GRAVES' DISEASE**—overactive thyroid gland.

>> **REACTIVE ARTHRITIS**—inflammation of joints, urethra, and eyes; may cause sores on the skin and mucus membranes.

>> **SJÖGREN'S SYNDROME**—destroys the glands that produce tears and saliva, causing dry eyes and mouth; may affect kidneys and lungs.

>> **TYPE 1 DIABETES**—destruction of insulin producing cells in the pancreas.

Unless you've been diagnosed with an autoimmune disease, the autoimmune epidemic is probably not on your radar screen. Especially since conventional medical thinking is that we have no idea what causes autoimmunity and that all we can do is utilize immunosuppressive medications.

That's not what the research shows, however. The research in this area is demonstrating that there are many avenues to explore in dealing with autoimmune disorders.

It basically comes down to making sure that every system of your body is operating as efficiently as possible. That is really the underlying strategy for all the areas of health and wellness that we are discussing in this book.

We're all at risk for autoimmune disorders. I believe that as the science and testing procedures advance, we're going to learn that the incidence of undiagnosed and more subtle autoimmune problems is much higher than we now realize.

Let's take a look at some autoimmune statistics for women, because women are three times more likely to get an autoimmune disease than are men. Recent statistics indicate that 9.7 million women are afflicted with one of the seven most common autoimmune disorders—lupus, scleroderma, rheumatoid arthritis, multiple sclerosis, inflammatory bowel disease, dry eye syndrome, or Type 1 diabetes. Women are five times more likely to have a serious, life-threatening autoimmune disorder than they are to have breast cancer or heart disease![33]

Unfortunately, if you have one autoimmune disorder, your risk of developing another is much greater. If you have even a mild autoimmune disorder such as dry eye syndrome, you're four times more likely to develop a more serious autoimmune disease in the future.[34]

The key to understanding autoimmunity is to look both broadly and specifically. Instead of waiting for definitive proof of a single cause of the condition, focus your energies on looking at broad health parameters. Do the obvious things first. If you have any problems at all with digestion, even subtle ones, focus on that first. That is so critical. Evidence suggests that an unhealthy gut may be the starting place of an autoimmune condition.[35]

Make sure your thyroid is functioning effectively and that your adrenal glands are working properly. Make sure that your circulation is good. Lower your cardiovascular risk factors as much as possible. Walking after meals is a powerful factor in dealing with autoimmunity. Don't think that just because you have an autoimmune disorder that you should be focusing on it to the exclusion of your overall wellness program.

Some studies have suggested that correcting an out-of-balance insulin level is a key strategy for anyone who has an autoimmune disorder or is at risk for one.[36] Insulin is one of the key hormones in the body. That's why when I wrote the book, *Goodbye Diabetes*, I felt that the title wasn't broad enough. It could have easily been titled, *Goodbye Disease*, because once you control insulin resistance, once you control excess production of insulin, you're doing what needs to be done to prevent and reverse chronic disease in general.

When insulin fluctuates dramatically throughout the day, as it does in prediabetes and diabetes, it magnifies fluctuations in other hormones, causing a variety of problems.

It's also very important to regulate cortisol in dealing with autoimmune disorders, because cortisol is related to adrenal health. Abnormal highs and lows of cortisol put your immune system at risk.[37, 38] But in order to stabilize cortisol, we must first prevent insulin spikes that occur after meals or snacks.

The immune system in your body is like a SWAT team that is ready to be called upon to come in and deal with an emergency. But when there is an autoimmune disorder in the body, it's as if the SWAT team has gone rogue and begins shooting peaceful citizens and blowing up innocent women and children! Our own immune system that was designed to protect us at all cost, becomes dysfunctional and begins destroying good and bad cells alike. When autoimmune disorders strike, we have to figure out their underlying triggers. Once we discover the various factors that cause autoimmunity, then we can develop a plan for helping the body to heal.

LATENT AUTOIMMUNE DIABETES

Type 1 diabetes usually develops rapidly due to an autoimmune disorder. However, about 20 percent of individuals with Type 2 diabetes actually have a much more slowly developing autoimmune disorder.[39, 40] The body can start producing antibodies against the insulin-manufacturing cells in the pancreas, thus damaging their ability to produce insulin, or it can produce antibodies against the insulin itself, preventing it from connecting to its receptor sites. Either disorder disrupts the body's ability to control blood sugars.

This latent autoimmune diabetes typically occurs in people thought to have Type 2 diabetes, because they are still producing insulin. The autoimmune process progresses gradually, potentially taking years to ultimately destroy the pancreatic cells that make insulin. In Type 1 diabetes this cell destruction can take place within days or weeks.

I once had a diabetic patient who was a wrestling coach at the high school level. He was extremely fit; he worked out three hours a day. He was so fit that his adult sons, one of whom was a martial arts cage fighter, couldn't keep up with him in his workouts. Yet this man had out-of-control diabetes.

A "normal" Type 2 diabetic who could do even a fourth of this man's daily exercise workout would have been able to reverse his diabetes with lifestyle changes. Yet this man—this fit wrestling coach who was working out three hours a day—was struggling to control his blood sugars. Clearly, this was not typical Type 2 diabetes; something else was going on. It turned out that this man had latent autoimmune diabetes of adulthood (LADA).

An Australian study some years ago identified five factors that increase the likelihood that those who appear to have regular Type 2 diabetes actually have a latent autoimmune form of the disease (LADA).[41] The five factors were:

1. Developing the disease after age 50.

2. Having the acute symptoms usually associated with Type 1 diabetes.

3. Having normal weight, i.e., not being overweight (a Body Mass Index of less than 25).

4. Having a personal history of autoimmune disorders such as rheumatoid arthritis or multiple sclerosis.

5. Having a family history of autoimmune disorders.

The study found that if an individual has at least two of these five factors, the likelihood that his or her diabetes is the autoimmune form of the disease (LADA) is 90 percent!

For individuals whose diabetes is autoimmune related, simply controlling blood sugars with medication or insulin isn't really addressing the problem. In fact, that is also true even for those with regular Type 2 diabetes. Medication doesn't adequately address the underlying issue of insulin resistance.

PROTECTING THE EPIGENOME

The key thing to understand is that everything we do has the potential to change our epigenome. Everything in our environment, the choices we make regarding diet and lifestyle, how we choose to feel and think about our experiences—all these things influence our genetic expression. Nutrigenomics is the power of food to alter our genetic expression. Every time we go to the supermarket to buy groceries, every time we order food in a restaurant, we should be thinking about how we want our genes to express themselves and what effect our food choices will have on our epigenome.

Chapter 7 focused on our attitudes and emotions. These are an important part of our exposome. Negative emotional baggage will create negative expression in the genes. All these things have an effect on the immune system and our risk factors for autoimmune disorders.

In 2008, the journal *Autoimmune Review* published a study which found that up to 80 percent of those diagnosed with autoimmune diseases reported experiencing an unusual amount of emotional stress before the onset of the disease.[42]

We all have too much stress in our lives. We need to find emotional balance. We need to establish boundaries so that we can separate certain times and certain areas of our lives from all the stresses and pressures of modern life. Somehow, we need to find a way to put the brakes on the out-of-control lifestyle and the emotional stress that is such a significant factor in causing autoimmune disorders.

Studies are beginning to recognize that treatment of autoimmune diseases should include stress management and behavioral intervention to prevent stress-related immune imbalances. Stress, along with infection, trauma, and toxins, is a trigger causing the immune system to become dysfunctional and spawn autoimmune disorders. Stress is one of the worst toxins affecting our bodies, and we must learn how to manage it.[43]

> No matter what stresses life places on us, we still can choose how we will respond to that stress. And that response is what makes all the difference in the world.

Hostility and anger are basically emotional forms of inflammation.[44, 45] If left unresolved, over time, they will result in physical inflammation, which is so detrimental to our health and wellness. The apostle Paul wrote, "Do not let the sun go down on your wrath."[46] This is good advice no matter what religion or philosophy you follow. If you allow yourself to go to bed upset and angry, that is a source of inflammation driving up your health risk for autoimmune diseases and other illness.

SOME CAUSES OF AUTOIMMUNE DISORDERS

When the immune system goes rogue and turns against the body it is supposed to protect, that usually means some toxic influence on the body is changing the way the immune system is relating to healthy tissues. These toxins could be coming from a low-grade, or even a high-grade, infection. The reason infections are bad for us is that they release toxins into the body.[47] The worse the infection, the more toxins it releases.

This is such a problem that biomedical engineers at the University of California at San Diego recently developed nanosponges that are 3,000 times smaller than red blood cells (RBCs) and can absorb membrane-damaging toxins produced by antibiotic resistant bacteria like MRSA. Mice treated with nanosponges after exposure to lethal doses of MRSA toxins had a 44 percent survival rate. Giving the mice nanosponges *before* the lethal exposure increased the survival rate to 89 percent.[48] This study underscores the importance of having practical, easy to use detoxification strategies that not only can save your life, but also limit the effect of toxins on autoimmune and other chronic diseases.

> Many of the toxins we are exposed to are coming from low-grade infections that we don't even notice, because we're not running a fever and we don't necessarily feel bad. We can have chronic, untreated low-grade infections for decades.

Because we aren't aware of them, it's hard to get a handle on these infections and the toxins they are releasing into the body. But they are a major issue. What can we do about them?

Vitamin D can effectively limit infections and the toxins they release. But there is some concern today about getting too much Vitamin D. Let me assure you that getting "too much" Vitamin D should not be a priority concern. We need to stop worrying about overdosing on Vitamin D and make sure, instead, that we are getting enough. That's where the health risks are—not getting enough Vitamin D.

Check your Vitamin D levels, preferably twice a year—in the spring and fall. Make sure your Vitamin D blood levels are at least 50 ng/mL but they don't need to be more than 100 ng/mL. Keep in the upper half of the normal range, and that can powerfully decrease your risk of autoimmune disorders[49] and almost everything else.

So the first step in fighting autoimmunity is addressing the issues of toxins, low-grade infections, and inadequate nutrients, especially Vitamin D.

GLORIA'S STORY

When Gloria first came to see me she was very stressed. She was working twelve-hour days and commuting nearly two hours each way! Outside of work, she had very little in her life. She was experiencing debilitating pain in her hands and arms and had been diagnosed with rheumatoid arthritis. She was concerned that this condition would become so bad she couldn't use her hands—and then she would be out of a job. There were likely some genetic factors at play in her case; her mother had had rheumatoid arthritis for many years.

At this point, Gloria had been taking Methotrexate for five years. Doctors had told her that medication was all she could do to address her rheumatoid arthritis. Now she decided that she needed to take a broad approach to her health using lifestyle medicine principles. During our first office visit, I spent an hour and a half with her, looking at her total health situation and determining those things that needed immediate attention.

She was extremely low in Vitamin D. Her DHEA hormone level was also very low.

There are many studies showing that optimizing DHEA levels brings about dramatic improvement in persons with autoimmune disorders.[50]

We found that Gloria had some thyroid problems, including autoimmune thyroiditis. We started treating that aggressively. We did a four-hour glucose tolerance test and learned that she had diabetes although she had been completely unaware of it. All the chronic inflammation she had been experiencing for many years was causing significant insulin resistance and erratic blood sugars.

One and two hours into the glucose tolerance test, Gloria had very high blood sugar levels, but by three and four hours after taking the glucose drink, her blood sugar had dropped very low. She went from prediabetes to diabetes to reactive hypoglycemia and adrenal fatigue. Both the high and low sugars significantly affected her immune system and made her more predisposed to autoimmune problems. We also addressed her constipation and digestive problems. We developed a plan for every single system that was out of balance.

"Now," I told her, "I want you to go back and talk to your rheumatologist about gradually adjusting your medications because of the lifestyle changes you're making." She promised that she would.

A month went by. She came to see me again. "I can't believe how much better I feel," she said. "My problems are 90 percent resolved!"

Again I suggested to her that she needed to coordinate with her rheumatologist. I emphasized that she couldn't just stop taking medications such as Methotrexate. It could trigger a rebound inflammatory response that could be worse than her inflammation had been even before she started the medication. Again, she assured me she would follow up with her rheumatologist.

Another month passed, and another. It had been three months now since Gloria began the lifestyle medicine program. She said, "The pain is gone. I don't hurt anywhere!"

Four months into the program, I said, "You're working with your rheumatologist, right? You're doing so well, I'm sure your rheumatologist could help you get off those medications entirely with good, careful medical supervision."

She looked a little sheepish and said, "I haven't been completely honest with you. I stopped all those medications before the first month of the program was up."

Now I don't think that was a good idea. I don't advise that. But Gloria's story is an example of how powerful lifestyle medicine can be in improving health.

> When a person faithfully follows the whole program and incorporates it all into their total approach to life and health, amazing transformations can take place.

Gloria so dramatically improved her health that she was able to get away with discontinuing all her previous medications without experiencing the reaction that might be expected—a rebound inflammatory condition. I still encouraged her to consult with her rheumatologist to make sure she was being managed properly. Gloria was so excited at the changes lifestyle medicine had made. She felt great and was able to function better than she had in over a decade.

MARY'S STORY

Mary came to see me because she had problems with blood flow in her legs. In fact, scans had shown that she had peripheral artery disease. She had blockage in the arteries in her legs that made her legs feel heavy. That suggested that there was probably something going on also in her heart and in her carotid arteries that was increasing her risk for heart attacks and stroke.

After six months, she was doing much better with blood flow to her legs. "But what about my rosacea?" she asked. She had deep pustule lesions on her cheeks, which I hadn't noticed because of her makeup. But when she took the makeup off, I could see the deep pustules associated with autoimmune rosacea.

"Why don't you tell me about your medical history?" I asked. "There must be something else going on that we haven't addressed yet."

"How far back do you want me to go?"

"Fifteen years," I told her.

She thought a minute. "Let's see. Did I have my gallbladder taken out more than fifteen years ago?"

I said, "You never told me your gallbladder was removed."

"You never asked," she responded.

Fair enough! We started treating her digestion issues, knowing that she had no gallbladder, and in a month her rosacea had disappeared. She had struggled with it for decades.

Fixing whatever is broken in any system of your body, especially digestion, is critical to providing the immune system with the nutrients that it needs to begin the healing process.

DRY EYE SYNDROME

So many people have this common autoimmune problem. It's considered a mild condition, but it can be severe at times. One day I was talking to a doctor friend about Dry Eye Syndrome and how these autoimmune problems respond to lifestyle changes. He said, "My wife should talk to you. She has Dry Eye Syndrome."

She did come to see me. She, too, had had her gallbladder removed. We treated her digestion issues aggressively, and within weeks her Dry Eye Syndrome was resolved. The lesson here is: don't be satisfied in treating the external when the problem is related to an internal issue. Try to determine the actual cause of the problem and address it.

MARK'S STORY

A neighbor of mine, Greg, who traveled frequently on business trips, had a friend, Mark, whom he saw only every few months when he traveled to that area. On one visit, Greg noticed how emaciated Mark appeared. He had lost a lot of weight. Greg told Mark, "Something is wrong. You've got to deal with this."

Mark said, "Well, I'm seeing a doctor who has finally diagnosed my problem as ulcerative colitis. He's given me some medicine and tells me that is all I can do for it. But I'm having frequent blood loss in my stool."

A month went by, and Greg told me about his friend, Mark. He said, "He's lost a total of twenty-five pounds, and he didn't have any spare weight to lose to begin with. And Mark told me that he's losing a lot of blood when he has a bowel movement. He's essentially given up. He feels there is nothing he can do."

Greg said, "Wes, would you be willing to call Mark? I'll cover the consultation fee. Just call him and talk to him. Maybe you can help him."

I don't do that kind of thing very often. It's risky, because people have to *want* to change if lifestyle medicine is to be effective. But as a favor to Greg, I called his friend, Mark. I recognized that we needed a full hour to discuss his situation. I wasn't interested in just asking Mark how he was doing and saying, "God bless you; I hope you get better." If I was going to be any help, I needed to take enough time to begin figuring out what was going on with Mark and how to address it.

As Mark and I talked, we discovered that he needed to have a major diet change. He needed to get off all gluten. He needed to get off all dairy. That was tough for him, because pizza was his favorite food. But Mark realized that sometimes you have to say no to things you really want to do in order to say yes to the very best things.[51]

> Sometimes we need to say no to things we really like to eat, because there's something far better that will come from limiting ourselves in that way.

Limitations in certain areas of our lives can result in healing and blessings in other areas. The important thing is to look at the big picture and make the right choices as we consider the limits we need to set. It all has to be reasonable. It has to be part of an overall plan.

So that's what Mark did. He fixed his digestion, which was really critical for him. He took the appropriate nutritional anti-inflammatory products. In no time at all he wasn't bleeding anymore when he had a bowel movement. He started to gain weight. His skin color normalized. He was able to go back to work and feel energetic. He had new hope. That's been several years ago, and Mark is still feeling great.

GOOD HEALTH DOESN'T JUST HAPPEN

So many people walk around thinking, *If only I knew what was wrong with me, I could fix it.* But they don't do anything to help them figure out what is wrong or how to fix it. You have to want to be involved. It doesn't just happen. You've got to want to be cured, and if you really want it, you'll act in a way that lets you figure out what's going on. If we will pay attention to our body and its needs, we can achieve significant healing.

You can choose to follow a new direction that will make all the difference in your life. But, in the end, only you can make that choice. No one else can make it for you.

CHAPTER SUMMARY

>> Our bodies were made to constantly recreate themselves at the cellular level.

>> Even bad news can become good news if it causes you to focus on lifestyle interventions that bring about transformational change.

>> Inflammation is a common factor in most chronic and acute disease.

>> Autoimmune disorders occur when the body's immune system attacks and destroys healthy body tissue by mistake.

>> Evidence suggests that an unhealthy gut may be the starting place of an autoimmune condition.

>> If you have one autoimmune disorder, your risk of developing another is much greater.

>> Optimizing blood levels of Vitamin D can powerfully decrease your risk of autoimmune disorders.

>> Stress, infection, trauma, and toxins are triggers that cause the immune system to become dysfunctional and spawn autoimmune disorders.

>> Knowing what gene mutations you have provides the opportunity to seek solutions that could dramatically alter your risk of future disease.

>> The key to wellness is to identify the lifestyle triggers that can powerfully silence disease-causing genes and effectively activate health-promoting genes.

>> Hemoglobin A1C is an easily measured form of Advanced Glycated Endproducts (AGEs) that are produced by sugar irreversibly glazing to proteins.

>> Our body is always recreating itself. So if we give our body what it needs, it can actually reverse the irreversible.

>> A significant reduction of dietary AGEs can be achieved by eating more legumes, vegetables, fruits, and whole grains—and by avoiding solid fats, fatty meats, and highly processed foods.

>> Setting limits in certain areas of our life can result in healing and blessings in other areas of our life.

ENDNOTES

1 Vasdev, S.; Gill, V.; Singal, P.; "Role of Advanced Glycation End Products in Hypertension and Atherosclerosis: Therapeutic Implications," *Cell Biochemistry and Biophysics,* (2007) 49(1):48-63.

2 Brownlee, M., "Advanced Protein Glycosylation in Diabetes and Aging," *Annual Review of Medicine,* (1995) 46: 223-234.

3 Brownlee, M.; Vlassara, H.; Cerami, A.; "Nonenzymatic Glycosylation Products on Collagen Covalently Trap Low-Density Lipoprotein," *Diabetes,* (1985) 34: 938-941.

4 Bangert, A.; Andrassy, M.; Volz, C.; et al.; "The Role of Receptor for Advanced Glycation End Products and Its Ligand High Mobility Group Box 1 in Autoimmune Myocarditis," *Journal of the American College of Cardiology,* (2014) 63(12 S): doi:10.1016/S0735-1097(14)60972-4.

5 Coughlan, Melinda T., et al., "Advanced Glycation End Products Are Direct Modulators of ß-Cell Function," *Diabetes,* October 2011; 60:10 2523-2532; doi:10.2337/db10-1033.

6 Schmidt, A. M.; Hori, O.; Brett, J.; Yan, S. D.; Wautier, J. L.; Stern, D.; "Cellular Receptors for Advanced Glycation End Products: Implications for Induction of Oxidant Stress and Cellular Dysfunction in the Pathogenesis of Vascular Lesions," *Arteriosclerosis, Thrombosis, and Vascular Biology,* (1994) 14:1521-1528.

7 Goldin, Alison; Beckman, Joshua A.; Schmidt, Ann Marie; Creager, Mark A.; "Basic Science for Clinicians: Advanced Glycation End Products: Sparking the Development of Diabetic Vascular Injury," *Circulation,* (2006) 114:597-605, doi:10.1161/CIRCULATIONAHA.106.621854.

8 Uribarri, Jaime, et al., "Advanced Glycation End Products in Foods and a Practical Guide to Their Reduction in the Diet," *Journal of the American Dietetic Association,* (2010) 110.6; 911-916.e12. PMC. Web. March 22, 2015.

9 Geberhiwot, T.; Haddon, A.; Labib, M.; "HbA1c Predicts the Likelihood of Having Impaired Glucose Tolerance in High-Risk Patients with Normal Fasting Plasma Glucose," *Annals of Clinical Biochemistry,*(2005) May; 42(Pt 3):193-195.

10 Khaw, Kay-Tee, et al., "Association of Hemoglobin A1c with Cardiovascular Disease and Mortality in Adults: The European Prospective Investigation into Cancer in Norfolk," *Annals of Internal Medicine,* September 21, 2004, Vol. 141, No. 6, 413-420.

11 Selvin, Elizabeth, et al., "Glycemic Control and Coronary Heart Disease Risk in Persons With and Without Diabetes. The Atherosclerosis Risk in Communities Study," *Archives of Internal Medicine,* (2005) 165:1910-1916.

12 Cowie, C., et al., "Full Accounting of Diabetes and Pre-Diabetes in the U.S. Population in 1988-1994 and 2005-2006," *Diabetes Care,* 32 (2009) 287-294.

13 Stratton, Irene, et al., "Association of Glycaemia with Macrovascular and Microvascular Complications of Type 2 Diabetes (UKPDS 35): Prospective Observational Study," *British Medical Journal,* 321.7258 (2000): 405-412.

14 Stirban, Alin, et al., "Vascular Effects of Advanced Glycation Endproducts: Clinical Effects and Molecular Mechanisms," *Molecular Metabolism,* (2014) vol. 3, issue 2, 94-108.

15 Uribarri, Jaime, et al., "Advanced Glycation End Products in Foods and a Practical Guide to Their Reduction in the Diet," *Journal of the American Dietetic Association,* 110.6 (2010): 911-916.e12. PMC. Web. March 22, 2015.

16 http://www.elements4health.com/apoe4-slows-brains-ability-to-eliminate-amyloid-beta-in-alzheimers.html

17 Henrichs, I.; Froesch, D.; Wolf, A. S.; Teller, W. M.; "Impact of Apolipoprotein E on Alzheimer's Disease," *Current Alzheimer Research,* (2013) 10 (8): 809-817.

18 http://www.netplaces.com/alzheimers/understanding-alzheimers-risks/genetic-risks-for-alzheimers.htm

19 Sardi, F., et al., "Alzheimer's Disease, Autoimmunity and Inflammation. The Good, the Bad and the Ugly," *Autoimmunity Reviews,* December 2011; 11(2):149-153. doi: 10.1016/j.autrev.2011.09.005.

20 Sneed, Annie, "DDT, Other Environmental Toxins Linked to Late-Onset Alzheimer's Disease," *Scientific American,* February 10, 2014.

21 Mishra, S.; Palanivelu, K.; "The Effect of Curcumin (Turmeric) on Alzheimer's Disease: An Overview," *Annals of Indian Academy of Neurology,* (2008) 11(1):13-19. doi:10.4103/0972-2327.40220.

22 Exley, Christopher, "Drinking Mineral Water Could Reduce Aluminum in Alzheimer's Disease Sufferers." "Non-Invasive Therapy to Reduce the Body Burden of Aluminium in Alzheimer's Disease," *Journal of Alzheimer's Disease,* vol. 10, no. 1, 17-24, September 2006. http://www.j-alz.com/vol10-1

23 Cardoso, B., "Importance and Management of Micronutrient Deficiencies in Patients with Alzheimer's Disease," *Clinical Interventions in Aging,* 8 (2013): 531-542. *PMC.* Web. March 29, 2015.

24 Carter, J., "Alzheimer's Disease: A Pathogenetic Autoimmune Disorder Caused by Herpes Simplex in a Gene-Dependent Manner," *International Journal of Alzheimer's Disease,* (2010), Article ID 140539, 17 pages. doi:10.4061/2010/140539

25 Letenneur, L., et al., "Seropositivity to Herpes Simplex Virus Antibodies and Risk of Alzheimer's Disease: A Population-Based Cohort Study," (2008) *PLoS ONE,* vol. 3, no. 11, Article ID e3637.

26 Itzhaki, R. F.; Wozniak, M. A.; "Alzheimer's Disease-Like Changes in Herpes Simplex Virus Type 1 Infected Cells: The Case for Antiviral Therapy," *Rejuvenation Research,* (2008) vol. 11, no. 2, 319, 320.

27 Bradley, H.; Markowitz, L. E.; Gibson, T.; McQuillan, G. M.; "Seroprevalence of Herpes Simplex Virus Types 1 and 2—United States, 1999-2010," *Journal of Infectious Diseases,* (2013) DOI: 10.1093/infdis/jit458.

28 Roberts, C. M.; Pfister, J. R.; Spear, S. J.; "Increasing Proportion of Herpes Simplex Virus Type 1 As a Cause of Genital Herpes Infection in College Students," *Sexually Transmitted Diseases,* (2003) 30:797-800.

29 Belshe, R. B.; Leone, P.A.; Bernstein, D. I.; et al.; "Efficacy Results of a Trial of a Herpes Simplex Vaccine," *New England Journal of Medicine,* (2012) 366:34-43.

30 Itzhaki, R. F; Dobson, C. B; Lin, W. R.; Wozniak, M. A.; "Association of HSV1 and Apolipoprotein E-ε4 in Alzheimer's Disease," *Journal of NeuroVirology,* (2001) vol. 7, no. 6, 570-571.

31 "MedlinePlus Medical Encyclopedia—Autoimmune Disorders," National Institutes of Health. July16, 2014. Retrieved December 21, 2014.

32 http://www.healthline.com/health/autoimmune-disorders#Overview1

33 Nakazawa, Donna Jackson, *The Autoimmune Epidemic* (New York, NY: Simon and Schuster, 2008).

34 Ibid.

35 Campbell, Andrew W., "Autoimmunity and the Gut," **Autoimmune Diseases,** (2014) 152428. PMC. Web. March 29, 2015.

36 Nokoff, N., "The Interplay of Autoimmunity and Insulin Resistance in Type 1 Diabetes," *Discovery Medicine,* February 14, 2012.

37 Derijk , R., "The Immune-Hypothalamo-Pituitary-Adrenal Axis and Autoimmunity," *International Journal of Neuroscience,* July 1991; 59(1-3):91-100.

38 Nutan, Kanwar A. J.; Bhansali, A.; Parsad, D.; "Evaluation of Hypothalamic-Pituitary-Adrenal Axis in Patients with Atopic Dermatitis," *Indian Journal of Dermatology, Venereology, and Leprology,* May-June 2011; 77(3): 288-293.

39 http://www.healthline.com/diabetesmine/all-about-lada

40 Latent Autoimmune Diabetes in Adults (http://www.annalsnyas.org/cgi/content/full/958/1/112); Mona Landin-Olsson; Department of Diabetology and Endocrinology, University Hospital, S-221 85 Lund, Sweden; *Annals of the New York Academy of Sciences,* (2002) 958:112-116.

41 Fourlanos, S.; Perry C.; Stein, M. S.; Stankovich, J.; Harrison, L. C.; Colman, P. G.; "A Clinical Screening Tool Identifies Autoimmune Diabetes in Adults," *Diabetes Care,* (2006) 29:970-975.

42 Stojanovich, L., "Stress as a Trigger of Autoimmune Disease," *Autoimmunity Reviews,* January 2008; 7(3):209-213. doi: 10.1016/j.autrev.2007.11.007.

43 Ibid.

44 Boisclair, Demarble J., "The Relation Between Hostility and Concurrent Levels of Inflammation Is Sex, Age, and Measure Dependent," *Journal of Psychosomatic Research,* May 2014; 76(5):384-393. doi: 10.1016/j.jpsychores.2014.02.010.

45 Miller, G., "Cynical Hostility, Depressive Symptoms, and the Expression of Inflammatory Risk Markers for Coronary Heart Disease," *Journal of Behavioral Medicine,* vol. 26, no. 6, December 2003.

46 Ephesians 4:26, NKJV.

47 Geerts, S., "Systemic Release of Endotoxins Induced by Gentle Mastication: Association With Periodontitis Severity," *Journal of Periodontology,* (2002) 73:1, 73-78.

48 Hu, Che-Ming, "A Biomimetic Nanosponge That Absorbs Pore-Forming Toxins," *Nature Nanotechnology,* (2013) 8, 336-340; doi:10.1038/nnano.2013.54.

49 Yang, C., "The Implication of Vitamin D and Autoimmunity: A Comprehensive Review," *Clinical Reviews in Allergy & Immunology,* October 2013; 45(2):217-226. doi: 10.1007/s12016-013-8361-3.

50 Sawalha, Amr H., Kovats, Susan, "Dehydroepiandrosterone in Systemic Lupus Erythematosus," *Current Rheumatology Reports,* (2008) 10.4: 286-291.

51 Paraphrased from Gordon MacDonald, *Ordering Your Private World.*

Playing with Poison

DETOXIFICATION FOR OPTIMAL HEALTH

WHEN I BRING UP THE SUBJECT OF DETOXIFICATION and health with patients, they often give me a strange look. Sometimes, they ask, "Why should we be considering how to detoxify our bodies? Doesn't the body just do that on its own?"

Yes, our bodies should be detoxifying themselves. But since 1945, following World War II, more than 100,000 new toxins have been developed and released into the environment.[1] Published reports suggest that of all these toxins that are currently on the market, less than 1 percent have been properly studied and evaluated regarding their impact on human health, and only a handful have been regulated. That's a problem! Today, we live in a new age—a new paradigm. In some ways, it's much harder today to achieve good health than it was in the past, simply because we're exposed to so many more toxic substances that can break down our health and limit our healing potential.

THE MAIN SOURCE OF TOXICITY

So let's look at the issue of toxicity. Where does it come from, and what can we do about it?

A major theme of this book has been the importance of understanding how to change our epigenome and the expression of our genes. We are all born with thousands of healthy genes, as well as thousands of genes that, potentially, predispose us to all kinds of disease, disability, and premature death. The most important factor for health and wellness is not whether we have those less-than-perfect genes; it's what we do with them. The totality of what we do with them is called our exposome. Our exposome is everything in our world, everything in our environment, everything that we eat, everything that we drink, everything that we think, everything that we do, the air we breathe, every activity that we're involved in—all this makes up our exposome. All these things affect our genes and their expression.

Most people don't realize that the majority of the toxins to which we're exposed come to us through our food. As we've seen throughout this book in many different contexts, the power of diet to alter our genetic expression is extremely significant. That's why it's so critical that we think about the foods we eat as we consider the issue of toxicity. What foods are most likely to bring with them the toxins that can weaken and tear down our body's systems?

THE DIRTY DOZEN AND THE CLEAN FIFTEEN[2]

The Environmental Working Group (EWG) publishes a list of produce containing the highest levels of pesticides. This list is known as the Dirty Dozen.™ EWG's *Shopper's Guide to Pesticides in Produce* recognizes that many people who want to reduce their exposure to pesticides in produce cannot find or afford an all-organic diet. The EWG guide helps them seek out conventionally grown fruits and vegetables that tend to test low for pesticide residues. Or if conventional versions test high for pesticides, individuals can make an effort to locate organic versions. The 2015 Dirty Dozen list (the produce with the worst levels of pesticides) is comprised of apples, peaches, nectarines, strawberries, grapes, celery, spinach, sweet bell peppers, cucumbers, cherry tomatoes, imported snap peas, and potatoes. Key findings:

» *99 percent of apple samples, 98 percent of peaches, and 97 percent of nectarines tested positive for a least one pesticide residue.*

» *The average potato had more pesticides by weight than any other produce.*

» *A single grape sample and a sweet bell pepper sample contained fifteen pesticides.*

» *Single samples of cherry tomatoes, nectarines, peaches, imported snap-peas, and strawberries showed thirteen different pesticides apiece.*

The EWG's Clean Fifteen™ list of produce *least* likely to hold pesticide residues consists of avocados, sweet corn, pineapples, cabbage, frozen sweet peas, onions, asparagus, mangoes, papayas, kiwis, eggplant, grapefruit, cantaloupe, cauliflower, and sweet potatoes. Relatively few pesticides were detected on these foods, and tests found low total concentrations of pesticides on them. Key findings:

» *Avocados were the cleanest. Only 1 percent of avocado samples showed any detectable pesticides.*

» *Some 89 percent of pineapples, 82 percent of kiwis, 80 percent of papayas, 88 percent of mangos, and 61 percent of cantaloupes, had no residue.*

» *No single fruit sample from the Clean Fifteen™ tested positive for more than four types of pesticides.*

Multiple pesticide residues are extremely rare on Clean Fifteen vegetables. Only 5.5 percent of Clean Fifteen samples had two or more pesticides. Visit ewg.org for more information and updates on the amount of pesticides in fruits and vegetables.

Dr. Michael Greger, M.D., of NutritionFacts.org is one of the world's leading educators regarding the impact that the foods we eat have on our health. "Let me make one thing clear," Dr. Greger states,[3] "even if you can't find organic options. So while organic is absolutely better, we should never avoid buying fruits and veggies out of fears of pesticide exposure. But if you have the choice and the means, certainly buy organic."

Ultimately, our goal is to eat lots of fruits and veggies while doing our best to limit our exposure to toxins of any kind. Remember, up to 90 percent of pesticides come from animal products—mainly dairy, meat and fish.[4]

FAST FOOD IS MOSTLY BAD FOOD

As we look at our exposome in terms of diet, there is good food and there is bad food. Fast food is mostly bad food. One reason is that fast food doesn't provide the nutrients we need. The healthy nutrients that we should be getting in our food are the sources of the chemicals that help neutralize toxins in our bodies. They prevent toxins from hooking up to enzymes, receptor sites, and to our genes, causing destruction and harm throughout our system.[5]

Another reason fast food is mostly bad food is that it brings with it toxins that have been introduced into it during the process of making it easy to prepare and more tasty. Healthful foods that come to us from nature—colorful, natural, whole-plant foods—function as antitoxins.

TOXICITY AND DIABETES

In 2006, several medical journals published findings from the National Health and Nutrition Examination Survey that was completed in 2002. The researchers took blood samples from 2,016 adult participants. Those with the highest concentrations of persistent organic pollutants (POPs) in their blood were thirty-eight times more likely to have diabetes. That's almost a 4,000 percent greater risk of being diabetic. Even those with less than average levels of toxins in their blood were still fourteen times more likely to have diabetes than those who had undetectable levels.[6]

In other words, having even some exposure to toxins increased the risk of having diabetes by 1,400 percent.

"Obesity was a risk factor for diabetes only if the people had blood concentrations of pollutants above a certain level. It was interesting that there was no association between obesity and diabetes among subjects with non-detectable levels of pollutants."[7]

This study strongly suggests that our focus should not be on weight loss but rather on avoiding the main sources of toxins and on eating more whole, plant-based foods that help the body detoxify. Ironically, this would also be the best way to lose weight. After learning about this study, I made sure that all my patients with diabetes or prediabetes were educated on effective detoxification strategies.

TOXINS MODIFY GENE EXPRESSION UP TO THE FOURTH GENERATION

We know that toxins can damage our DNA, leaving us with mutated genes that are passed on to our children. But now we are learning that the effect of toxins can be passed on up to four generations—all the way to our great grandchildren—even though the toxins didn't cause mutations to our genes. The damage from the toxin is done by altering the DNA methylation pattern and therefore affecting which genes are turned on or turned off.

> Here lies another example of how we control not only our epigenetic destiny, but also the epigenetic destiny of the three generations that come after us—our great-grandchildren!

In 2005, Dr. Michael Skinner, a biology professor at Washington State University, reported that exposure of pregnant rats to a fungicide caused reduced sperm counts as well as significantly impaired sperm motility in the next three generation of males—even though all three subsequent generations of rats were never exposed to the fungicide toxin.[8] Dr. Skinner has also shown that without changing or mutating the genetic code, a toxic exposure to our great-grandmother could powerfully affect our risk of many conditions, including high cholesterol, kidney disease, prostate problems, and immune system abnormalities. One of *Discover* magazines top stories of 2007 was how three consecutive generations of male rats, born to a female exposed to fungicide, were consistently rejected by potential female partners.[9]

More recently, "short-term exposure of pregnant rats to several kinds of chemicals caused ovarian disease not just in their daughters, but also in two subsequent generations of females." Exposure to "fungicide, pesticides, dioxin, jet fuel, and a mixture of plastics" produced symptoms similar to human polycystic ovarian syndrome and ovarian insufficiency.[10] This syndrome is also strongly associated with headaches, infertility, and increased risk of heart disease, diabetes, and cancer.[11] This is the amazing new field of epigenetic transgenerational inheritance. More sobering is the fact that our children and their grandchildren may inherit, not just our genes but also the expression of our genes as determined by what we eat, drink, think, how we behave, and how we interact with the world around us. On the bright side, this also means that we can make the lives of our grandchildren much better by educating our children about the power of epigenetic inheritance.

THE PROBLEM OF MERCURY AND ARSENIC IN FOOD

The majority of toxins we are exposed to in our food supply does not come from pesticides on fruits and vegetables. The main source of environmental toxins comes from eating food that has been building up toxins during its entire lifetime. Consider the buildup of mercury in fish. Isn't it sad that a food that historically has been healthful—especially for island cultures—has become so toxic?

> It's difficult today to find fish that aren't loaded with mercury. That's why even the U.S. government warns women who are pregnant or breast-feeding not to eat fish more than once or twice a week.

Now, if the government warns you not to eat something, you can be sure there is a problem! The government is frequently the *last* organization to tell you not to eat something. That is because there is so much vested interest in the status quo, so many lobbyists for various food industries, that politicians are reluctant to rock the boat. That's also the reason the war on obesity has shifted its focus almost entirely from diet to exercise. Don't misunderstand. Exercise is good for us and important for many reasons. But what we eat has a much bigger influence on obesity and our risk for disease than does exercise. Food has such a powerful influence on our health that it's imperative for us to understand what foods are best for us.

Why is there so much mercury in fish today? Here is what is happening. Little fish eat plants and tiny little organisms in the ocean that have been exposed to the mercury fallout caused by burning coal all around the world as well as other sources. Then slightly bigger fish come along and eat the little fish. In one or two bites, they consume all the mercury that the little fish has accumulated in its body during its entire lifetime. Then an even larger fish eats that fish—and consumes all the mercury that fish has taken in from all the little fish it has eaten. You get the picture. We call this process, bio-magnification. The largest fish, the ones we humans tend to eat, are now seriously high in mercury.

Mercury in the food we eat is a crucial issue.[12] Mercury is a neurotoxin.[13] Between 1980 and the year 2000, Alzheimer's exploded twofold[14] and is projected to double again by 2025.[15] As rates skyrocket, we're trying to come to grips with all the factors that might be related to this growing problem. Scientific reports continue to point to micronutrient deficiencies[16] [17] and toxicity in our environment as key factors in the increased incidence of Alzheimer's and dementia.[18, 19, 20]

In a large Southern California study, individuals consuming meat, fish, and poultry were twice as likely to develop dementia compared to vegetarians and three times more likely to do so if they had regularly consumed meat, fish, and chicken for many years.[21] Avoiding the main sources of toxins while emphasizing plant-based foods that are rich in nutrients is a powerful combination in the prevention and even the reversal of cognitive decline. A 2014 study conducted by the UCLA Center for Alzheimer's Disease Research showed that when a comprehensive lifestyle medicine approach was provided to patients with Alzheimer's, 90 percent showed improvement in memory within three to six months of starting the program.[22]

What other foods are loaded with toxins? I'd like to suggest that any animal we eat has been "bio-magnifying" toxins its entire life.[23] The amount depends, of course, on what food that animal has consumed.[24] Many are aware that mercury and other toxins accumulate in fish, but most are unaware that the majority of chickens are actually given feed that has arsenic added to it because of its antibiotic effects. At least 75 percent of Americans eat chicken on a regular basis, most of which has unacceptably high levels of arsenic.[25]

"Chronic inorganic arsenic exposure has been shown to cause lung, bladder, and skin cancers and has been associated with other conditions as well, including heart disease, type 2 diabetes, cognitive deficits, and adverse pregnancy outcomes."[26] We need to look carefully at the food we eat. We need to understand where the toxins are coming from so that we can make good choices. We need to effectively weigh the benefits and the risks. We need to consider the many components of our exposome, and then ask ourselves this question: "What parts of my lifestyle expose me to toxins that will negatively affect my epigenome and therefore how well my genes function?"

TOXICITY AND HEART DISEASE

Another underlying concern throughout all the areas we have been discussing in this book is the issue of inflammation. Anytime you are exposed to a toxin, that toxin is going to create inflammation.[27]

The number one killer among adults around the world is cardiovascular disease, which is primarily an issue of toxicity.[28]

The degree of inflammation in the body can change quickly from day to day and week to week. For individuals who have risk factors for heart disease, these changes in inflammation are something they need to monitor routinely and pay attention to. Plaque can build up inside the artery walls very quickly. It doesn't have to take years or decades to develop. It may develop slowly, but it can build up in a matter of weeks, depending on what's going on inside the artery wall itself.[29, 30] For instance, serious infections[31] and poisonous spider bites release toxins that can promote rapid buildup of artery plaque.[32]

Blood levels of environmental toxins found in elderly individuals are directly related to the level of plaque buildup in their arteries.[33] All this strongly suggests that both the level and the number of different toxins we are exposed to influence not only our risk of disease but also how quickly disease develops.

The good news is that by understanding the factors that trigger and prevent arterial plaque buildup, we can also develop strategies to reverse it.[34] In fact, more than fifteen years ago, Dr. Dean Ornish clearly demonstrated that coronary disease is very much reversible by following a comprehensive lifestyle medicine program.[35]

Today there is an advanced test for cardiovascular risk that is part of the Hunter Heart Profile.[36] This particular test is the Lp-PLA2 test,[37] often referred to informally as the "PLAC" test.[38] It monitors for the release of an enzyme in the blood that comes primarily from foam cells—the cells inside the artery wall that are forming plaque.[39] It's important to have this test, because if you have this problem, you should want to know about it. You need to know in order to take whatever steps are necessary to reverse the plaque buildup. Whenever there is a problem in the body, there is always a cause-and-effect relationship. So once you determine your risk, you can do the detective work. You can figure out what is causing inflammation inside the vascular bed of the artery wall and promoting the buildup of plaque.[40] Once you know the cause, you can begin working to treat it.

> The best science right now tells us that heart disease, or atherosclerosis, begins when various forms of toxin are introduced into the arterial wall.[41] The toxins then get into the cholesterol and turn it into aggressive, inflammatory particles that attract white blood cells.

As the white blood cells come flooding in to try to clean up that toxic area, they ingest so many toxic cholesterol particles that they form into foam cells, like slimy Styrofoam pellets that clump together into larger plaques that build up in the artery wall, thus narrowing the space for blood flow. Since that's how the process works, and since it begins with a toxin, maybe we should be giving some thought to where those toxins came from. Maybe we should be asking how we can decrease the amount of toxins getting into the bloodstream and artery wall.

When it comes to cardiovascular disease, I believe there are two main factors that are driving this condition—toxins and infections. However, they get very little attention clinically. Low-grade infections actually create a toxic environment in the bloodstream that increases inflammation and therefore speeds up plaque formation. This is especially evident with low-grade, chronic dental infections, even when there are no symptoms.[42]

Since heart disease is strongly related to some type of exposure to toxins, we need to reason from cause to effect to figure where these toxins are coming from and how we're being exposed to them. We need to monitor our lab tests and use the results to help us know where to focus our attention. See chapter 12 for more information on lab testing.

THE VALUE OF KNOWING YOUR RISK FACTORS

The ApoLipoprotein E (ApoE) test, as we've seen before, can be a valuable tool to evaluate the risk for heart disease,[43] plaque buildup, and especially for Alzheimer's disease.[44] In the previous chapter, we saw that if you have two mutated copies of this Apo E gene, your risk for Alzheimer's goes up as much as 34-fold.[45] That's more than 3,000 percent! But understanding this risk doesn't mean that you have to accept the consequences. Instead, it means that now you have some information that you can use to alter that future destiny. Understanding our risk for these things lets us do something about it and negates much of that risk by further evaluating the possible triggers and then aggressively dealing with each of them.

If we have these gene mutations or other risk factors, it means that we're more predisposed to these toxins that influence our health. It means that some of us need to be far more careful than others with what we allow into our exposome.

It's easy to think, *If she can eat that, I should be able to as well.* But we know that isn't really true. When it comes to health, comparing ourselves to other people doesn't work very well, because we're all so genetically and biochemically different. We're biologically unique.

So avoid comparing yourself to others. The only person you should compare yourself to is YOU.

Someone you think is fit and healthy might actually be must less healthy than you! Some individuals go around saying, "My cholesterol is only 150." Because their cholesterol is so low, they assume they are really healthy, when that may not be the case at all. Health or wellness is not determined by one or two or even ten different risk factors. It's determined by the big picture.

More important, good health is advanced by being willing to look for our weaknesses—so we can address their root causes. Human nature naturally drives us to emphasize our strengths and shy away from our weaknesses. We may even not want to know what our weaknesses are. But careful monitoring and prompt attention to problems will save you immense amounts of misery and health challenges later on.

DETOXIFICATION AND HEALING

How can paying attention to the process of detoxification help you achieve optimal wellness?

For decades, Dr. Sidney Baker was a professor at Yale University Medical School and a family physician. After retirement, he began thinking about what he had learned in medical school and what he had taught medical students through the years. He realized there were some things he hadn't appreciated sufficiently at the time. So he wrote a book, *Detoxification and Healing*.[46] Here is one statement from that book:

"Illness and disease will affect the body's detoxification chemistry, and if there's something wrong with detoxification, any other health problem will be aggravated."

He's saying that no matter what genetic predispositions you may have, if your body has a problem removing toxins, you're in trouble. You're not going to be able to achieve optimal wellness. That's why it is so important to detoxify your body.

> Toxicity integrates with everything else that is going on in your body and affecting your health. Your immune system, digestion, and circulation—all these important areas are key elements in the process of detoxification. They are all interrelated.

So optimal health and the potential to heal requires that we provide all the necessary elements and remove any interfering elements. These are the two key aspects of any wellness program, of any healing program. Nutrients are the necessary elements for optimizing the system. That's the way it's always been. Without these necessary elements your body can't heal.[47]

Eating a healthy diet isn't primarily about optimizing weight or lowering your cholesterol or even lowering your blood sugars. Primarily, it's really about giving your body the very building blocks by which it can heal. That's the bottom line. But it doesn't stop there. Nutrients are the necessary elements for healing, but toxins are the interfering elements.

> Optimal health requires not only that we provide the body with all the necessary elements to support its function; but also requires that we eliminate interfering elements—the toxins that tear down the body and destroy health.

ENVIRONMENTAL TOXINS, ENDOGENOUS TOXINS, AND ENDOTOXINS

It's also important to recognize that toxins aren't just things that come to us from the outside. We refer to these as *environmental* toxins. Included in the category are persistent organic pollutants (POPs), pesticides, herbicides, fungicides, and heavy metals like mercury, lead, and arsenic.

A second group of toxins are *endogenous* toxins. These are internally generated toxins produced as the natural byproduct of respiration, digestion, metabolism, and the body's breakdown and repair processes. These are the toxins and waste products that even a healthy body produces minute by minute and day by day. If we are alive, our body is producing endogenous toxins. The body is constantly taking in oxygen and removing carbon dioxide. If it can't do so, the carbon dioxide becomes toxic.[48] The kidneys are constantly removing toxins that are a natural byproduct of metabolizing food and breaking down protein.

A third class of toxins are *endotoxins* that come from within the bacteria when they die and disintegrate. As bacteria are killed by our immune system or by antibiotics, they can release large amounts of endotoxins resulting in symptoms such as high fever, chills, inflammation, muscle and joint pain, fatigue, headache, and anxiety. When released in large amounts, endotoxins can cause severe symptoms often referred to as the "die-off reaction." The scientific term for this is the "Herxheimer Reaction," named after Dr. Karl Herxheimer,[49] a German-Jewish dermatologist who first described this process in 1902.[50] More recently, the Herxheimer reaction to endotoxins has been described in *The Lancet* [51]and *The New England Journal of Medicine.*[52]

The body is actually designed to effectively and efficiently neutralize toxins and then remove them. So we should be trying to understand how this works and how we can help the body do its job well. The best way to help the body naturally detoxify itself is to make sure that every system of the body is working efficiently.

GENETIC INDIVIDUALITY, SUSCEPTIBILITY TO TOXINS, AND VITAMIN C

Everyone is biologically different and genetically unique. Each of us is "one-of-a-kind." We each have distinctive strengths and weaknesses, specific susceptibilities, and peculiar predispositions. Two-time Nobel laureate, Dr. Linus Pauling, one of the brightest scientists of the twentieth century, said that "each person's health benefits from having the right molecules in the right amounts."

Our body was designed to work best when getting the optimal variety and amounts of many nutrients.

Dr. Pauling had the uncanny ability to look at a problem and understand it at its deepest levels. Some people are like that. They just know. In science, Dr. Pauling was one of those individuals. Yet some in scientific circles derided him for saying that we should have more of the healing elements in our bodies and focus more on taking in nutrients that can protect our DNA, optimize the function of our genes, support the immune system, and neutralize toxins. "The standard American diet," his critics argued, "provides all the nutrients necessary for good health."

I would argue that the standard American diet is responsible for many forms of micronutrient deficiency and malnutrition. It is also responsible for exposing us to a toxic load that powerfully promotes disease and creates a barrier to healing. I would also argue that now, more than ever, we need to eat an optimal, plant-based diet because of current agricultural standards, our genetic susceptibility, and our exposure to many sources of toxins (including emotional and non-diet-related sources). In addition, each of us would benefit from developing a prudent, individualized, and evidenced-based supplemental nutrient support program.

Let's look at an example of how optimizing one single nutrient can overpower the otherwise devastating effects of a genetic mutation. A study published in 2010 by the Federation for American Societies of Experimental Biology dealt with Werner's Syndrome, a genetic disease that causes rapid aging.[53] People with this disorder begin to show signs of accelerated aging in their 20s. They develop age-related diseases and generally die before the age of 50.

This study showed that Vitamin C stopped and even reversed accelerated aging in a group of mice that had the genetic mutation causing Werner's Syndrome. These mice had become fat, diabetic, and were rapidly developing hair loss, heart disease, osteoporosis, cataracts, and cancer. That's a bad combination. When they were given extra Vitamin C in their drinking water, these mutated mice improved their ability to burn fat and experienced decreased tissue inflammation and oxidative stress. After treatment with Vitamin C, they became as healthy and lived as long as the non-mutated mice.

But we don't have to have a rare genetic mutation to suffer from premature aging. Bacterial endotoxins can cause the same damaging inflammation and oxidative injury in anyone. Dr. Archie Kalokerinos, a physician in Australia, has written extensively on the therapeutic effect of Vitamin C on endotoxins.[54] He has also successfully used Vitamin C injections to reduce the risk of sepsis caused by potentially lethal levels of endotoxins released by dying bacteria or parasites. Higher levels of endotoxins significantly decrease Vitamin C in the blood and cells,[55] requiring a much higher intake of this nutrient.[56][57]

The point is that many risk factors, including gene mutations and toxin exposure, create a much higher necessity for key nutrients.

Please don't misunderstand. I'm not saying that all your problems will be solved if only you take enough Vitamin C. That's not the case. But it is certainly true that we need to understand what factors are promoting unhealthful levels of inflammation and oxidative stress and therefore predisposing us to premature disease and disability. We should look for the answer in the two basic factors determining wellness: (1) Are we being exposed to all the necessary nutrients we need for our given genetic tendencies? (2) As far as possible, are we removing unnecessary exposure to the toxins that greatly increase our need for those very nutrients? See chapter 12 on how genetic testing can help us determine our unique nutritional needs.

SYMPTOMS VERSUS CAUSES

It's important to understand that so much of healthcare today focuses on treating symptoms instead of treating the cause. Dr. Sidney Baker, the author of *Detoxification and Healing,* illustrated this point with what he called the "thumbtack rule." "If you're sitting on a tack," he said, "it takes a lot of aspirin to make you feel good."[58]

> What's the obvious approach to solving the problem of sitting on a thumbtack? Do you focus on the symptom and treat your pain with aspirin? Or does it make more sense to fix the cause of the problem by getting up and removing the tack?

Dr. Baker went on to make an even more telling point. He said, "If you're sitting on *two* tacks, removing just one doesn't result in a 50 percent improvement." That's an important principle. So often, I've heard people say, "Yes, I tried going on a healthful diet, and I felt worse." Or they say, "I tried exercising, and it didn't work. My blood sugars went up when I started exercising; I'm never going to do that again." What do such statements suggest? They indicate that the person was unwilling to follow through and do whatever was necessary to optimize healing.

Is it possible that someone could switch to a plant-based diet and feel worse? Of course! You need to act wisely and thoughtfully when you make any lifestyle change. You may need to counsel with individuals who understand these issues and who can guide you successfully. Sometimes you need to have somebody walk you through these strategies, because there is so much going on in your body that when you make one good change, it can backfire somewhere else.

That can happen especially if you are taking medications when you begin making lifestyle changes. When you start eating better and exercising more often, for example, your need for blood pressure medications or blood sugar medications can drop quickly. If you are not working with your physician to appropriately adjust your medications as you start making these positive, healthy decisions, you could begin feeling a lot worse, because now you're over-medicated. You could even end up in the emergency room, trying to figure out why you're doing so poorly. In such cases, it's easy to blame it all on the diet and exercise program, when in fact those are the things that are making you so healthy you no longer need as much medicine!

> The answer is to pay attention and be proactive about adjusting your medicines with the help of your doctor when you begin to make significant lifestyle changes.

ENDOTOXINS FROM OUR FOOD

Endogenous toxins are formed as the natural byproduct of respiration, digestion, metabolism, and the body's breakdown and repair processes. But as we discussed above, endotoxins are somewhat different, because these toxins come from within the bacteria when they die and disintegrate. When we consume animal products the endotoxins that were generated from bacteria in the animal's body now become *extra* endotoxins that affect us directly. The high heat of cooking may kill the bacteria, but it also liberates the endotoxins which are unaffected by cooking.

In 2009, Dr. Ghanim, from the University at Buffalo, conducted a clever experiment. He fed individuals two styles of breakfast. One group ate 910 calories from an egg muffin, sausage muffin sandwiches, and two hash browns. The other group also ate 910 calories, but this time the calories came from fruit and fiber-rich breakfast foods including oatmeal, milk, orange juice, English muffins, peanut butter, and raisins. Dr. Ghanim checked everyone's blood levels before eating and again at one, two, and three hours after eating. The study found that eating the "adult happy meal breakfast" with the eggs, cheese, and sausage, caused a rapid transfer of the animal-generated endotoxins directly into the bloodstream. This transfer of endotoxins was further promoted by the increased amounts of animal fats in the meal. These endotoxins quickly stimulated the release of inflammatory chemicals, promoted resistance to insulin, abnormally increased blood sugars, and turned up oxidative stress reactions. The harmful changes lasted for three hours, but were totally absent after eating the fruit and fiber-rich breakfast.[59]

A 2010 study evaluated how a 300-calorie drink of cream, glucose, or orange juice affected blood levels of endotoxins, inflammation, and oxidative stress. The glucose drink, like any pure sugar drink, was free of endotoxins, but still increased levels of inflammation in the blood. Amazingly, the orange juice (OJ) had five times more endotoxins than did the cream. Pasteurization of partially spoiled OJ kills the bacteria, but not the endotoxins! But ingesting the OJ did not raise blood levels of endotoxins at all. The many plant-based nutrients in the OJ and the absence of animal fat in the drink completely prevented the transfer of the endotoxins from the digestive system into the bloodstream. Even though the OJ was loaded with 300 calories of fruit sugar, there was no increase in inflammation or oxidative stress. Compared to the OJ, the cream drink had a much lower level of endotoxins. But the cream's high fat content and lack of protective plant nutrients led to a 17 percent increase of endotoxins in the subjects' circulating blood. The cream also increased all the measures of inflammation and oxidative stress. This increase started within one hour of drinking the cream and lasted for five hours! This study demonstrates that animal fat intake and inadequate nutrients are key contributors to inflammation and disease-promoting pathology in our bloodstream.[60]

Another study showed that those with prediabetes or diabetes had much higher baseline values of circulating endotoxins. Even before eating the high-animal-fat breakfast, diabetic individuals had 60 percent higher levels of endotoxins in their blood than did the non-obese control participants who did not have diabetes. After the high fat meal, the diabetics' endotoxin levels were higher for the next four hours and 125 percent higher than the control group a full four hours after the meal.[61] In other words, being overweight, prediabetic, or having other health concerns makes us especially vulnerable to toxins. These studies demonstrate that the foods we eat have the ability to generate healing or to produce disease and disability. Ultimately, what we eat on a regular basis is a matter of life and death.

TOXINS AND ACTIVATED CHARCOAL

About twenty years ago in California, a woman moved some boxes as she was cleaning her garage. As she did so, a spider bit her on the arm. She was soon in tremendous pain. She went to her doctor. Her doctor determined that she had been bitten by a Brown Recluse spider. At that time there was no known antidote. The standard treatment was to cut out tissue from around the bite surgically, hoping to remove some of the venom that was extremely toxic. So that is what her doctor did.

But the toxins from the spider bite kept spreading and spreading. The woman began having terrible pain and poor circulation throughout her arm. Within a week, she was experiencing chest pains. Further evaluation showed that she had developed significant plaque buildup in the arteries of her heart. This was someone who had no known risk factors for heart disease prior to the spider bite. Atherosclerosis and coronary heart disease can develop within a few weeks if you're being exposed to a significant toxin[62] or infection.[63]

This woman ended up having heart surgery two weeks later. But she could have potentially avoided all that if she had been aware of the healing properties of something as simple as activated charcoal. If she had made a little poultice of activated charcoal with flaxseed oil or extra virgin olive oil and promptly placed it over the area of that spider bite and changed it every couple of hours, she could have potentially resolved her problem within days.

> The medicinal value of activated charcoal should be considered in any look at detoxification.

If I could take only one medicinal product with me to an undeveloped part of the world where infectious diseases and intestinal illnesses were prevalent,

I would take activated charcoal powder. I would take as much of it as I could. It's inexpensive, and it has multiple uses both externally and internally.

Some years ago our family was visiting relatives in Ohio when my youngest daughter, Katie, came down with intestinal flu. I knew she would be fine if I could get some activated charcoal. I went to a local pharmacy; the pharmacist there had never heard of activated charcoal. I went to another, and that pharmacist knew nothing about it either. Finally, I went to a third, larger, pharmacy. "Yes," the pharmacist said, "I know about activated charcoal, but we don't have any. That's old folk medicine. We have much better medications now."

I beg to disagree.

> In my experience, nothing is more effective for intestinal flu or other intestinal infections than activated charcoal. No companies market it, however, because it's so inexpensive and there is little money to be made. That is unfortunate because it could save families from significant medical bills as well as from the misery of being up all night with intestinal flu.

Let me tell you a trick about how to use it. Ten years ago, while living on the beautiful island of Guam, I came home late one evening, and my wife greeted me at the door with the news that our daughters, Madison and Katie, were sick. "Their tummies don't feel good," she said. "There has been some kind of bug going around the neighborhood, and now they appear to have it."

I looked at the girls; they were hunched over and had a sick look on their faces. Their eyes said, "We don't know what's wrong; just fix us!"

"Don't worry, girls," I said. "Daddy is going to make you a black shake."

They weren't too sure about that. The "shake" part sounded good, but they weren't too keen on it being black!

Madie, being the oldest and the most curious, followed me to the kitchen and watched as I scooped up a heaping teaspoon of charcoal. By the way, always do this over the sink, because the charcoal powder is so fine it will go everywhere if you're not careful! Fill a glass half full with cold water and put it in the sink. Then carefully transfer the charcoal powder to the glass and mix it thoroughly. If you leave even a little film of charcoal on the surface of the water, it will go right into your lungs when you take that little breath you always take just before the first sip. If that happens, it's not the end of the world, but you don't want to be coughing for the next couple of minutes.

As Madie watched me mixing up the charcoal "shake," she said, "Oh, Daddy, that doesn't look very good."

Instantly, I realized my mistake. I shouldn't have let her watch me make it. And instead of using a clear glass, I should have put it in a carton or a colored cup, with a dark straw, so she wouldn't have noticed that it was black and yucky looking.

Thinking quickly, I said, "Oh, honey, this isn't for you! This is for me. I don't want to get sick like you." And I proceeded to drink the entire black shake.

She watched me drink it all. Then she asked, "Well, what about me?"

"Oh! Would you like some, too?"

Of course, she would. So I made another one just for her. I made sure the water was very cold. That's the trick. Use cold water and add ice cubes. Mix it thoroughly with a heaping teaspoon of charcoal. If it's *really* cold, it tastes almost minty. I don't know how else to describe it. But if you use regular tap water, it will taste like chalk water. It won't be very tasty!

Katie came into the kitchen while her big sister was drinking the black shake. So, of course, she wanted to have one too. Within thirty minutes, both girls were feeling fine! They slept soundly all night, and Mom and Dad didn't have to get up four or five times in the night to help two little vomiting girls.

Fast forward about three years. We were now living in Southern California, and Katie was now 8 years old. Again, I came home one evening to find that Katie wasn't feeling good. I looked her over, but I wasn't paying much attention. She looked okay. So we all went to bed. About 2:30 in the morning I sensed a presence hovering over me. I awoke to find Katie leaning over my bed, her long, stringy hair tickling my face. She was staring down at me. "Daddy," she managed to say, "I don't feel good. I'm going to throw up!"

I jumped out of bed and rushed her to the bathroom. I was holding her hair out of her face as she retched into the toilet! "Daddy," she gasped, "can you make me a black shake?"

At 2:30 in the morning, while vomiting and feeling terrible, she knew the antidote. She knew exactly what she needed, because she had experienced the benefit three years earlier.

I made both of us a black shake and made sure she drank it all. I put her back to bed. She fell asleep within minutes and slept the rest of the night. I also got to sleep the rest of the night!

My daughter Madie has enjoyed participating in mission trips to undeveloped areas of Mexico, Peru, and the Philippines. Every time she has gone, she has asked me for a full thirty-two-ounce container of activated charcoal powder. I don't have to encourage her. She just knows that charcoal is her best bet to keep from getting sick. She takes a little each day and a full "black shake" if she feels she has been exposed. Many of Madie's friends kid her about her nasty-looking remedy. But she has never gotten sick, and before the end of the mission trip most of her friends have come to her, eager to cure their intestinal misery with doses of Madie's "black shake." On two extended mission trips everyone got sick except Madie.

That's the medical value of charcoal. Everyone should have a large container of activated charcoal powder as the most important part of their home medical emergency kit.

The benefits of charcoal remind me of a popular American Express slogan—"Don't leave home without it." I know Madie never will.

NATURAL DETOXIFYING STRATEGIES

There are many detoxifying strategies that utilize natural means. Some of my favorites include sauna therapy and any form of hydrotherapy using alternating hot and cold water treatments. Some cultures around the world have taken advantage of this strategy on a regular basis as a way to improve general well-being.[64] There is something amazingly therapeutic about heating your body to the point that you're beginning to get uncomfortable, then immediately taking a really cold shower or plunging into a frozen lake or ocean or into a pool of cold water, and then returning to the heat.[65]

If you take the time to do some hot/cold/hot/cold therapy at the first sign of a cold or flu, or any kind of an infectious sickness, it can dramatically boost the effectiveness of your immune system, and it will increase white blood cell leukocytes as well as the number and activity of natural killer cells that are key in fighting viral infections and cancer.[66, 67] You will feel a lot better after doing hot/cold therapy. It can be as simple as going into your shower and gradually turning up the water temperature until it is as hot as you can take it on your chest and throat.

Of course, be sure to regulate the temperature carefully so that you don't burn yourself! Let the hot water run three or four minutes and then turn it all the way cold. You can also place a shallow pan of ice right outside the shower. After standing under the hot water, rub ice on your chest and throat for about thirty seconds, and then go back to the hot water for three or four minutes, and repeat three times. It will invigorate your immune system tremendously. Saunas and hot therapies create a sweat, and every time you sweat you release toxins.[68]

Bringing yourself to a sweat every day, either through exercise or hot/cold therapy, is a good practice.

I spent some time in Finland recently. I was intrigued by the sauna houses built right on the shore of the Baltic Sea. While I was there, a family who had a sauna in their home invited me to enjoy it. After sitting in the hot sauna, we walked out on the ice of the Baltic Sea and took a plunge into the ocean through a hole in the ice. It was like jumping into a giant Slurpee! Basically, like an "ice-bucket challenge" on steroids!

When we came out of the water, we sat on their porch for ten minutes or so in the freezing weather—and we didn't feel cold! We repeated the steam sauna process and what I called the "Finnish Slurpee Plunge" several times and experienced a natural "runner's high" from the release of endorphins. It was a beautiful experience. And in the process we were optimizing our immune function and detoxifying.[69] Even toxic heavy metals are removed from our body when we have a good sweat.

ADDITIONAL TESTS FOR TOXICITY

There are various laboratory tests that may be useful by helping us find the "gaps" in our detoxification process. The "gaps" are areas of concern that are currently not being addressed in our personal wellness program. Whether it's an unintended exposure, an inherited genetic defect, or a greater need for specific nutrients, knowing our specific "gaps" can guide us in developing the right therapeutic strategies. In this section I briefly review a few of the tests that may help your doctor answer these questions. This is by no means a comprehensive list. Some of these tests are beneficial for everyone, while others are needed only by those with specific symptoms or concerns. Chapter 12 goes into much more detail on some of these tests.

Ferritin. A key test that I believe everyone should get is one that measures your iron levels and especially the storage form of iron called ferritin. If your body has a tendency to store iron in the form of ferritin, it gradually becomes toxic to your body, increasing whatever risk you already have toward heart disease,[70] diabetes,[71] cancer,[72] and many other conditions.[73] It's a simple thing to measure, but it isn't usually included in a standard physical. It's important to know if you have an iron overload problem, because that can cause a heart attack, diabetes, retinal detachment, or other complications all by itself.

Ammonia. Other tests related to detoxification look at ammonia levels in the body. If they are abnormal, there are nutritional strategies for dealing with the problem.

Liver Enzymes. Testing liver enzymes is another area to consider. If your liver enzymes are high, that means your liver, the main detoxification organ, is struggling. What is the liver supposed to be doing? It's supposed to be going through Phase I and Phase II detoxification, and if it can't do that effectively, cells inside the liver start dying much too quickly. When these cells die, they release their enzymes. Elevated levels of liver enzymes indicate that liver cells are dying more rapidly than normal. This test is clearly something we need to pay attention to.

Glutathione. When clients have unexplained fatigue or tend to get sick easily, I often have them get their blood tested for glutathione levels. When glutathione levels in the blood become low, it is a strong indication that the body, especially the liver, is struggling to neutralize and remove toxins.

Glutathione is one of the body's most important antioxidants for neutralizing free radicals, boosting the immune system, and optimizing the liver's detoxification function. If glutathione levels are below normal, it is important to work with a nutritionally savvy health professional to get this resolved.[74]

Homocysteine. A blood test for homocysteine is also important in detoxification. When homocysteine builds up in the blood it becomes mildly toxic to many body systems. Optimal levels are less than 7.2. Levels above 9.0 are strongly suggestive of a functional Vitamin B12 insufficiency and possibly of an inadequate intake of Folate and Vitamin B6.

Homocysteine is an amino acid that is converted into cysteine from methionine. When the converting enzymes have inadequate access to the activating vitamins, homocysteine will accumulate to unhealthy levels. Elevated homocysteine indicates increased irritation and a system-wide inflammation that promotes resistance to normal thyroid function in spite of normal thyroid levels on lab tests. Higher than optimal levels of homocysteine are associated with increased risk of heart disease,[75] Alzheimer's, dementia, depression, osteoporosis, kidney disease, certain cancers, and many other health concerns.[76, 77] Elevated homosysteine levels can also impair the body's ability to repair itself after an injury or surgery.

Regular intake of meat products stimulates excess production of homocysteine. And coffee, in particular, increases homocysteine. Limiting or completely avoiding coffee is one way to lower this risk factor.

Additional reasons homocysteine may be elevated include use of antacid medications, oral contraceptives, estrogen use, inadequate production of stomach hydrochloric acid at meal time (hypochlorhydria), and *H. Pylori* bacterial infection in the stomach. Even when homocysteine levels are not elevated, it is also a good idea to check for the MTHFR gene mutation which is associated with a much greater need for methyl folate and vitamin B12. The MTHFR gene mutation test can detect a genetic mutation which limits the body's ability to activate the vitamin folate, and that means your body can't detoxify itself well.[78]

Mercury and Lead. I once had a patient in Guam who owned a jewelry store at a local tourist mall. She was very health conscious. She ate lots of vegetables. She stayed away from meat. She ate fish. She was trying to do everything she could to be healthy. All the same, she suffered from chronic fatigue.

It just so happened that about the time she came to see me, I had just read an article by Dr. Jane Hightower, an internist in San Francisco, who had had a very similar case. The patient in the article exercised daily, ate well, but was becoming increasingly fatigued. Her internist was sharp. She didn't just keep repeating the same tests. She began studying, trying to understand what was going on with this woman. That's the kind of doctor you want, if you have a health problem—someone who will study your condition and not just do the same standard things he or she does for everyone.

> Your doctor needs to study your unique condition to figure out specifically what is going on that is influencing your health negatively.

Finally, the internist suggested testing her patient's blood levels for mercury, because her symptoms indicated she might be mercury-toxic even though she didn't have any significant exposure to mercury at home or work. Levels of mercury should be at least below 5 mcg/L. But any detectable level represents a potential health risk. A week later, when the test results arrived, the physician's concerns were validated as the mercury level was very high at 26 mcg/L. Dr. Hightower's diagnosis was chronic, low-level mercury poisoning.

As the internist evaluated the patient's diet, she learned that because the woman was avoiding red meat and even chicken, she was eating more of her favorite fish—mackerel. Mackerel is a fish that happens to be quite high in the food chain, meaning that it has a significant biological accumulation and bio-magnification of mercury. Eliminating fish from her diet brought the patient's mercury levels down to normal, but it took a year.

I had read this article, so when my patient came with a similar complaint I suggested we check her mercury level. It was 46—almost twice as high as the patient in San Francisco that had made international news! I asked about her diet and learned that she liked fish. But almost everybody in Guam eats fish. My experience on Guam, of testing most of my patients for mercury, taught me that if they ate two or more servings of fish per week, their levels of mercury would be 10 or higher. So I thought, *Diet can't be the only thing that is going on here.* I began asking more questions. Then a thought came to me. She was selling jewelry at her kiosk. And mercury is used in manufacturing the kind of inexpensive costume jewelry she sold. Every day she would grab a little ring and show it to someone, put it back, and pick it back up again later. She was constantly touching these rings and bracelets that were contaminated with mercury.

Can you actually get mercury toxicity by handling jewelry made with mercury? Absolutely! You can develop lead toxicity by carrying around lead pipes. I've seen it in several of my patients. Handling lead pipes or any lead based item without gloves will transfer small amounts of lead into your bloodstream. Whatever you touch can get into your blood. In fact, anything you put on your hands or on your body gets into your blood, too.

We need to be aware of the things to which we're exposing ourselves. So pay attention to the lotions, cosmetics, make-up, and household cleaning products you use. If you have health problems, it may be wise to use environmentally safe cosmetics and non-toxic brands of household products.

Magnesium. Magnesium is another lab test we should consider. Magnesium is a healing nutrient that directly influences many, critical body function. The vast majority of adults in the United States are low in magnesium,[79] and if you have diabetes, prediabetes, heart disease, or hypertension, chances are your magnesium levels are even lower than average.[80] That scenario creates a perfect environment for mercury to take over. One of the reasons mercury is toxic is because if interferes with cellular functions by attaching to where magnesium is supposed to be.[81] You should be paying attention to your magnesium levels.

Kidney Function. Kidney function is crucial to detoxification. Filtering and detoxifying of blood is the primary function of our kidneys. Healthy kidneys filter out waste products and toxins from the seven to eight liters of blood in our bodies—not just once a day, but twenty-five times every day! It they aren't functioning efficiently, we are going to have a toxicity problem. See chapters 8 and 12 for more information on kidney function and testing.

Hormones. Hormone panels can be of value as well. Abnormal levels of certain hormones can reflect health risk for various diseases. When managing certain health conditions, it may be helpful to determine if your hormones are being properly detoxified by the liver.[82] Many hormones can also be easily tested using saliva samples.

IDENTIFYING AND ADDRESSING YOUR NEEDS

Make sure your healthcare team is helping you tailor a program that helps you identify weaknesses and problem areas in your health. Detoxification involves many systems and organs in the body.

In this chapter you have learned that the combination of your total "toxic load," your daily intake of nutrients, and your genetic individuality, together determine your ability to optimize detoxification and therefore your potential for health and healing. By applying these concepts intentionally and proactively you have the opportunity to dramatically transform your health.

CHAPTER SUMMARY

>> The majority of toxins to which we are exposed come to us through our food.

>> "Fast food" is mostly bad food.

>> The Dirty Dozen™ is a list of the twelve fruits and vegetables that contains the highest levels of pesticides.

>> The Clean Fifteen™ is a list of the fifteen fruits and vegetables least likely to hold pesticide residues.

>> Eating high on the food chain leads to significant accumulation and bio-magnification of toxins.

>> Up to 90 percent of our dietary pesticide exposure comes from eating meat, chicken, fish, eggs, and milk.

>> Exposure to toxins prior to having children can affect the health of your children, grandchildren, and even your great-grandchildren.

>> Risk for headaches, infertility, heart disease, diabetes, and cancer can result through epigenetic transgenerational inheritance from as far back as your grandparents.

>> Having two mutated copies of the Apo E gene increases your risk for Alzheimer's as much as thirty-four-fold. Most of this risk can be reversed.

>> UCLA provided a comprehensive lifestyle medicine approach for patients with Alzheimer's, and 90 percent of them showed improvement in memory within three to six months of starting the program.

>> Toxins in the body are a major cause of inflammation and oxidative stress.

>> Cardiovascular disease, the number one cause of death worldwide, is primarily an issue of toxin-induced inflammation in the arteries.

>> At least 75 percent of Americans eat chicken on a regular basis, most of which has unacceptable levels of arsenic.

>> Sources of toxins include environmental toxins (pesticides, herbicides, fungicides, and heavy metals like mercury, lead, and arsenic), endogenous toxins (internally generated toxins produced as the natural byproduct of body metabolism), and endotoxins (toxins released from within the bacteria when they die and disintegrate.

>> Saunas, hot/cold therapies, and exercise promote sweating. Every time you sweat you release toxins.

>> Healthcare today often focuses on treating symptoms instead of treating the cause.

>> Thumbtack Rule #1: If you're sitting on a tack, it takes a lot of aspirin to make you feel good.

>> Thumbtack Rule #2: If you're sitting on two tacks, removing just one doesn't result in a 50 percent improvement.

>> Everyone should have a large container of activated charcoal powder as an important part of their home medical emergency kit. It's cheap, practical, and a very effective detoxifying agent.

ENDNOTES

1 https://www.scribd.com/doc/120627547/Introduction-from-Toxicants-Health-and-Regulation-since-1945

2 The material in this section is taken largely from The Environmental Working Group's website—ewg.org.

3 http://nutritionfacts.org/video/nine-servings-a-day-minimum/

4 http://www.peta.org/living/food/meat-contamination/

5 Ambrosone, C. B.; Tang, L., "Cruciferous Vegetable Intake and Cancer Prevention: Role of Nutrigenetics," *Cancer Prevention Research*, (Philadelphia, PA) April 2009; 2 (4): 298-300.

6 Lee, D., "A Strong Dose-Response Relation Between Serum Concentrations of Persistent Organic Pollutants and Diabetes: Results From the National Health and Examination Survey 1999-2002," *Diabetes Care*, July 2006; 29 (7): 1638-1644.

7 Porta, Miquel, "Persistent Organic Pollutants and the Burden of Diabetes," *The Lancet*, vol. 368, no. 9535; 558-559, August 12, 2006.

8 Anway, Matthew D.; Cupp, Andrea S.; Uzumcu, Mehmet; Skinner, Michael K., "Epigenetic Transgenerational Actions of Endocrine Disruptors and Male Fertility," *Science*, June 3, 2005: 308 (5727), 1466-1469. [DOI:10.1126/science.1108190].

9 Crews, David; Gore, Andrea C.; Hsu, Timothy S.; Dangleben, Nygerma L.; Spinetta, Michael; Schallert, Timothy; Anway, Matthew D.; Skinner, Michael K.; "Transgenerational Epigenetic Imprints on Mate Preference," *Proceedings of the National Academy of Sciences*, (2007) 104 (14) 5942-5946; published ahead of print, March 26, 2007, doi:10.1073/pnas.0610410104.

10 http://www.motherjones.com/blue-marble/2012/06/can-exposure-toxins-change-your-dna

11 Nilsson, E.; Larsen, G.; Manikkam, M.; Guerrero-Bosagna, C.; Savenkova, M. I.; et al., "Environmentally Induced Epigenetic Transgenerational Inheritance of Ovarian Disease," *PLoS ONE*, (2012) 7(5): e36129. doi:10.1371/journal.pone.0036129.

12 Castoldi, A., "Neurotoxic and Molecular Effects of Methylmercury in Humans," *Reviews on Environmental Health*, (2003) January-March; 18 (1):19-31.

13 Lucchini, R., "Neurotoxic Effect of Exposure to Low Doses of Mercury," *Medicina del Lavoro*, (2002) May-June; 93 (3):202-214.

14 Hebert L. E.; Scherr, P. A.; Bienias, J. L.; et al., "Alzheimer Disease in the U.S. Population: Prevalence Estimates Using the 2000 Census," *Archives of Neurology*, (2003) 60:1119-1122.

15 American Health Assistance Foundation (AHAF): About Alzheimer's Disease Information page. Available at: http://www.ahaf.org/alzdis/about/adabout.htm. [Accessed 2005.]

16 Cardoso, B., "Importance and Management of Micronutrient Deficiencies in Patients with Alzheimer's Disease," *Clinical Interventions in Aging*, (2013) 8:531-542. doi: 10.2147/CIA.S27983. Epub May, 10 2013.

17 Lopes da Silva, S.; et al., "Plasma Nutrient Status of Patients with Alzheimer's Disease: Systematic Review and Meta-Analysis," *Alzheimers & Dementia*, July 2014: 10(4):485-502. Epub October 19, 2013.

18 Farina, M., "Mechanisms of Methylmercury-Induced Neurotoxicity: Evidence from Experimental Studies," *Life Sciences,* (2011) 89:555-563.

19 Olivieri, G., "Mercury Induces Cell Cytotoxicity and Oxidative Stress and Increases Beta-Amyloid Secretion and Tau Phosphorylation in SHSY5Y Neuroblastoma Cells," *Journal of Neurochemistry,* (2000) 74:231-236.

20 Mutter, J., "Mercury and Alzheimer's Disease," *Fortschritte der Neurologie Psychiatrie,* (2007) 75:528-540.

21 Giem, P.; Beeson, W. L.; Fraser, G.; "The Incidence of Dementia and Intake of Animal Products: Preliminary Findings from the Adventist Health Study," *Neuroepidemiology,* (1993) 12(1):28-36.

22 Bredesen, D., "Reversal of Cognitive Decline: A Novel Therapeutic Program," *Aging,* (Albany, NY) 6.9 (2014): 707-717.

23 Chelsea, M., "Ingested Plastic Transfers Hazardous Chemicals to Fish and Induces Hepatic Stress," *Scientific Reports,* 3, Article number: 3263 doi:10.1038/srep03263. Published November 21, 2013.

24 Bhupander, Kumar, "Bioaccumulation of Heavy Metals in Muscle Tissue of Fishes from Selected Aquaculture Ponds in East Kolkata Wetlands," *Annals of Biological Research,* (2011) 2 (5): 125-134.

25 Nachman, K. E.; Baron, P. A.; Raber, G.; Francesconi, K. A.; Navas-Acien, A.; Love, D. C., 2013. "Roxarsone, Inorganic Arsenic, and Other Arsenic Species in Chicken: A U. S.-Based Market Basket Sample," *Environmental Health Perspectives,* (2013) 121:818-824; doi:10.1289/ehp.1206245.

26 Poultry Drug Increases Levels of Toxic Arsenic in Chicken Meat. http://www.jhsph.edu/news/news-releases/2013/nachman_arsenic_chicken.html

27 Lu, L, "The Inflammatory Heart Diseases: Causes, Symptoms, and Treatments," *Cell Biochemistry Biophysics,* February 15, 2015. [Epub ahead of print.]

28 "Optimizing Patient Cardiovascular Care with the Hunter Heart Profile," a 2014 presentation by Paul Ziajka, M.D., Ph.D., Director of The Florida Lipid Institute; Diplomat of the American Board of Clinical Lipidology; President of the South East Lipid Association.

29 von der Thüsen, Jan H.; van Berkel, Theo J. C.; Biessen, Erik A. L.; "Induction of Rapid Atherogenesis by Perivascular Carotid Collar Placement in Apolipoprotein E–Deficient and Low-Density Lipoprotein Receptor–Deficient Mice," *Circulation,* (2001) 103: 1164-1170; doi: 10.1161/01.CIR.103.8.1164.

30 Siess, Wolfgang; et al., "Lysophosphatidic Acid Mediates the Rapid Activation of Platelets and Endothelial Cells by Mildly Oxidized Low Density Lipoprotein and Accumulates in Human Atherosclerotic Lesions," *Proceedings of the National Academy of Sciences of the United States of America* (1999) 96.12; 6931-6936.

31 Headley, Adrienne J., "Necrotizing Soft Tissue Infections: A Primary Care Review," *American Family Physician,* July 15, 2003; vol. 68, no. 2.

32 Dean, Steven M., "Atypical Ischemic Lower Extremity Ulcerations: A Differential Diagnosis," *Vascular Medicine,* (2008) 13: 47-54.

33 Lind, P. Monica, "Circulating Levels of Persistent Organic Pollutants (POPs) and Carotid Atherosclerosis in the Elderly," *Environmental Health Perspectives,* (2012) 120:38-43 http://dx.doi.org/10.1289/ehp.1103563 [online October 11, 2011].

34 Kalanuria, Atul Ashok, "The Prevention and Regression of Atherosclerotic Plaques: Emerging Treatments," *Vascular Health Risk Management,* (2012) 8:549-561. Published online September 25, 2012; doi: 10.2147/VHRM.S27764.

35 Ornish D.; et al., "Intensive Lifestyle Changes for Reversal of Coronary Heart Disease," *Journal of the American Medical Association,* (1998) 280 (23):2001-2007. doi:10.1001/jama.280.23.2001.

36 http://hunterheart.com/hunterheart2.html

37 Kolodgie, F. D.; Burke, A. P.; Skorija, K. S.; et al., "Lipoprotein-Associated Phospholipase A$_2$ Protein Expression in the Natural Progression of Human Coronary Atherosclerosis," *Arteriosclerosis, Thrombosis, and Vascular Biology,* (2006) 26(11): 2523-2529.

38 http://www.plactest.com/healthcare/basic-science.html

39 Goldstein, L.B.; Bushnell, C. D.; Adams, R. J.; et al., "Guidelines for the Primary Prevention of Stroke: A Guideline for Healthcare Professionals from the American Heart Association/American Stroke Association," *Stroke,* (2011) 42:517-584. On behalf of the American Heart Association Stroke Council, Council on Cardiovascular Nursing, Council on Epidemiology and Prevention, Council for High Blood Pressure Research, Council on Peripheral Vascular Disease, and Interdisciplinary Council on Quality of Care and Outcomes Research.

40 Greenland, P.; Alpert, J. S.; Beller, G. A.; et al., "2010 ACCF/AHA guideline for Assessment of Cardiovascular Risk in Asymptomatic Adults: a Report of the American College of Cardiology Foundation/American Heart Association Task Force on Practice Guidelines," *Journal of the American College of Cardiology,* (2010) 56(25):e50-e103.

41 Ross, R., "Atherosclerosis—an Inflammatory Disease," *New England Journal of Medicine,* (1999) 340:115-126.

42 Cotti, E., et al., "Can a Chronic Dental Infection Be Considered a Cause of Cardiovascular Disease? A Review of the Literature," *International Journal of Cardiology,* (2010), doi:10.1016/j.ijcard.2010.08.011.

43 Lehtinen, S.; Lehtimaki, T.; Sisto, T.; et al., "Apolipoprotein E Polymorphism, Serum Lipids, Myocardial Infarction, and Severity of Angiography Verified Coronary Artery Disease in Men and Women," *Atherosclerosis,* (1995) 114:83-91.

44 Henrichs, I.; Froesch, D.; Wolf, A. S.; Teller, W. M., "Impact of Apolipoprotein E on Alzheimer's Disease," *Current Alzheimer Research,* (2013) 10 (8): 809-817. http://www.netplaces.com/alzheimers/understanding-alzheimers-risks/genetic-risks-for-alzheimers.htm.

45 Henrichs, I.; Froesch, D.; Wolf, A. S.; Teller, W. M., "Impact of Apolipoprotein E on Alzheimer's Disease," *Current Alzheimer Research,* (2013) 10 (8): 809-817.

46 Baker, S. M., *Detoxification and Healing,* Revised 2nd edition, (Chicago, IL, McGraw Hill, 2003).

47 Cardoso, B., "Importance and Management of Micronutrient Deficiencies in Patients with Alzheimer's Disease," *Clinical Interventions in Aging,* (2013) 8:531-542. doi: 10.2147/CIA.S27983. Epub May 10, 2013.

48 http://www.cdc.gov/niosh/idlh/124389.html

49 http://en.wikipedia.org/wiki/Karl_Herxheimer

50 Herxheimer, K.; Krause, D.; (1902). "Ueber eine bei Syphilitischen vorkommende Quecksilberreaktion," *Deutsche Medizinische Wochenschrift,* 28 (50): 895-897. doi:10.1055/s-0028-1139096.

51 "The Jarisch-Herxheimer Reaction," *The Lancet,* 1 (8007): 340, 341. February 1977. PMID 64863.

52 Fekade, D.; et al., "Prevention of Jarisch-Herxheimer Reactions by Treatment with Antibodies Against Tumor Necrosis Factor Alpha," *The New England Journal of Medicine*, August 1, 1996; 335 (5): 311-315. doi:10.1056/NEJM199608013350503. PMID 8663853.

53 Massip, L.,"Vitamin C Restores Healthy Aging in a Mouse Model for Werner Syndrome," *FASEB Journal*, January 2010; 24:158-172. http://www.fasebj.org/content/24/1/158.full

54 Kalokerinos, Archie, "Endotoxin and Vitamin C: Part 1—Sepsis, Endotoxin and Vitamin C," *Journal of the Australian College of Nutritional & Environmental Medicine*, April 2005; vol. 24, no. 1; 17-21.

55 Voigt, K., et al., "Decreased Plasma and Cerebrospinal Fluid Ascorbate Levels in Patients with Septic Encephalopathy," *Free Radical Research*, July 2002; 36(7):735-739.

56 Pleiner, J., et al, "High Doses of Vitamin C Reverse Escherichia Coli Endotoxin-Induced Hyporeactivity to Acetylcholine in the Human Forearm," *Circulation*. September 17, 2002; 106(12):1460-1464.

57 Armour, J., et al., "Ascorbate Prevents Microvascular Dysfunction in the Skeletal Muscle of the Septic Rat," *Journal of Applied Physiology*, March 2001; 90(3):795-803.

58 Baker, S. M., *Detoxification and Healing*, Revised 2nd edition, (Chicago, IL, McGraw Hill, 2003).

59 Ghanim, Husam, "Increase in Plasma Endotoxin Concentrations and the Expression of Toll-Like Receptors and Suppressor of Cytokine Signaling-3 in Mononuclear Cells After a High-Fat, High-Carbohydrate Meal—Implications for Insulin Resistance," *Diabetes Care*, December 2009; 32(12): 2281–2287. Published online September 15, 2009. doi: 10.2337/dc09-0979.

60 Deopurkar, R., "Differential Effects of Cream, Glucose, and Orange Juice on Inflammation, Endotoxin, and the Expression of Toll-Like Receptor-4 and Suppressor of Cytokine Signaling-3," *Diabetes Care*, May 2010; 33(5): 991-997.

61 Harte, Alison L., "High Fat Intake Leads to Acute Postprandial Exposure to Circulating Endotoxin in Type 2 Diabetic Subjects," *Diabetes Care*, February 2012; vol. 35, no. 2; 375-382.

62 Dean, Steven M., "Atypical Ischemic Lower Extremity Ulcerations: A Differential Diagnosis," *Vascular Medicine*, (2008)13:47-54.

63 Headley, Adrienne J., "Necrotizing Soft Tissue Infections: A Primary Care Review," *American Family Physician*, July 15, 2003; vol. 68, no. 2.

64 Huttunen P, Kokko L, Ylijukuri V. Winter swimming improves general well-being. Int J Circumpolar Health. 2004;63:140–4.

65 Mooventhan, A.; Nivethitha, L., "Scientific Evidence-Based Effects of Hydrotherapy on Various Systems of the Body," *North American Journal of Medical Sciences*, (2014): 6.5 199-209. PMC. Web. April 6, 2015.

66 Brenner, I. K.; Castellani, J. W.; Gabaree, C.; Young, A. J.; Zamecnik, J.; Shephard, R. J.; et al., "Immune Changes in Humans During Cold Exposure: Effects of Prior Heating and Exercise, *Journal of Applied Physiology*, (1999) 87:699-710.

67 Ring, J.; Teichmann, W., "Immunological Changes During Hydrotherapy," *Deutsche Medizinische Wochenschrift*, (1946) [1977, 102(45):1625-1630].

68 Genuis , S., "Blood, Urine, and Sweat (BUS) Study: Monitoring and Elimination of Bioaccumulated Toxic Elements," *Archives of Environmental Contamination and Toxicology*, August 2011; 61(2):344-357. doi: 10.1007/s00244-010-9611-5.

69 Crinnion, W. J., "Sauna as a Valuable Clinical Tool for Cardiovascular, Autoimmune, Toxicant-Induced and Other Chronic Health Problems," *Alternative Medicine Review*, (2011) 16:215-225.

70 Ellervik, C.; et al., "Total and Cause-Specific Mortality by Moderately and Markedly Increased Ferritin Concentrations: General Population Study and Metaanalysis," *Clinical Chemistry*, (2014) v. 60, 1419-1428. Published August 25, 2014.

71 Kunutsor, S., "Ferritin Levels and Risk of Type 2 Diabetes Mellitus: An Updated Systematic Review and Meta-Analysis of Prospective Evidence," *Diabetes/Metabolism Research and Reviews*, May 2013; 29(4):308-318. doi: 10.1002/dmrr.2394.

72 Alkhateeb, A., "The Significance of Ferritin in Cancer: Anti-Oxidation, Inflammation and Tumorigenesis," *Biochimica et Biophysica Acta*, December 2013; 1836(2):245-254. doi: 10.1016/j.bbcan.2013.07.002. Epub July 25, 2013.

73 Breimer, L., "Is Ferrotoxicity a New Great Public Health Challenge?" *Clinical Chemistry* (2015) v. 61, 667, 668. Published February 2, 2015.

74 Nuttall, S.; Martin, U.; Sinclair, A.; Kendall, M., 1998. Glutathione: In Sickness and in Health," *The Lancet* (1998) 351(9103): 645, 646.

75 Elizabeth, A., "Homocysteine and MTHFR Mutations: Relation to Thrombosis and Coronary Artery Disease," *Circulation*, (2005) 111:e289-e293; doi:10.1161/01.CIR.0000165142.37711.E7.

76 Alessandra, F. Perna, "Possible Mechanisms of Homocysteine Toxicity," *Kidney International*, (2003) 63, S137–S140.

77 Seshadri, S., et al., "Plasma Homocysteine as a Risk Factor for Dementia and Alzheimer's Disease," *New England Journal of Medicine*, (2002) 346: 476-483.

78 Elizabeth, A., "Homocysteine and MTHFR Mutations: Relation to Thrombosis and Coronary Artery Disease," *Circulation*, (2005) 111:e289-e293; doi:10.1161/01.CIR.0000165142.37711.E7.

79 Ervin, R., "Dietary Intake of Selected Minerals for the United States Population: 1999-2000," *Advance Data*, April 2004; 27; (341):1-5.

80 Del Gobbo, L., "Circulating and Dietary Magnesium and Risk of Cardiovascular Disease: A Systematic Review and Meta-Analysis of Prospective Studies," *American Journal of Clinical Nutrition*, July 2013; 98(1): 160-173.

81 Milosević, M., et al., "Effects of Metal Ions on Plasma Membrane Mg2+-atpase in Rat Uterus and Ovaries," *Annals of the New York Academy of Science*, June 2005; 1048: 445-448. PubMed PMID: 16154973.

82 Schneider, J., et al., "Abnormal Oxidative Metabolism of Estradiol in Women with Breast Cancer (Endogenous Estrogens/16a-hydroxylation/Endocrine-Related Tumors)," *Proceedings of the National Academy of Sciences*, USA, May 1982; vol.79, 3047-3051.

—ELEVEN—

Rest is Best

How Sleep Impacts
Your Health

As I work with patients and hold health and wellness seminars, people often ask, "Of all the health strategies we've been discussing and learning about—which is the most important?"

I usually smile and answer, "The most important health strategy for you is the one you're not following!"

If you're neglecting or overlooking a particular strategy for optimizing your health, you're not only depriving yourself of the benefits of that particular strategy, you're also not taking advantage of the synergy that comes from the interaction between all the components of a comprehensive wellness program. Every time you add one more effective approach to the list of wellness strategies you're implementing, you get an exponential increase in healing potential because of the synergy effect.

IS THERE ONE KEY HEALTH STRATEGY?

But setting all that aside for a moment, is there a single health strategy that is more important than any other, and if so, what would it be?

Would it be good nutrition? Nutrition is clearly a powerful influence on the body. What about regular exercise? Exercise is so critical and makes such a tremendous impact on health. Hydration? How long can a person survive without water? Not long. It may be possible, in certain environments and circumstances, to survive up to two weeks without water. But even a day without water significantly compromises our health. Proper hydration is essential to our physical existence and well-being. How about the lack of sunlight or Vitamin D? Its lack dramatically increases our risk for disease. Perhaps the most important wellness strategy is avoiding such things as smoking or alcohol or other substances that create stress and a toxic condition in the body. Finally, what about daily exposure to fresh air, proper rest and sleep, or forgiveness and trust?

All of these wellness strategies seem to be so critical, so essential. But is there one that is key to making all the others successful? Is there one that, if forgotten and neglected, will largely keep us from benefiting from the others?

That is an important question, because as we have seen throughout this book, health and wellness is a matter of overall, integrated epigenetic change—the power of your exposome to influence and change the expression of your genes. It's not a matter of isolated, unrelated health strategies. It's a holistic, integrated program that includes everything in and around you that determines the function of your genes and therefore the path that takes you on the journey towards either health of disease. So what is it that sets the stage for you to be willing and able to follow all these health strategies and benefit from them?

For example, we've looked at the power of nutrition and nutrigenomics—the powerful influence of food on our genes. But what leads us to make poor dietary choices? Is it simply lack of willpower? I don't think so. It's not so much a lack of willpower as it is a lack of effective planning, a lack of awareness regarding the subtle factors that ultimately determine whether we will make good choices today, tomorrow, and next week—whether we will be able to maintain and continue an effective wellness program. We know the power and benefit that is in colorful, whole, plant-based foods. We know that it's the colors, the pigments themselves, in these foods that can change the expression of our genes. But what enables us *to choose* to follow a first-class diet?

As we saw in Chapter 7, our very thoughts and attitudes can powerfully alter our genes in many ways. But what is it that causes us to be irritated, hostile, cynical, and angry? What is going on in our lives that makes it so difficult to control our thoughts and attitudes?

We come back to the question: Is there a single health strategy that is key to making all the others successful?

ADEQUATE SLEEP IS THE KEY

Even back when I was a freshman in high school, I really cared about my health. I thought a lot about it and about how I could be as healthy as possible. I had read in the book, *Ministry of Healing*,[1] about eight laws of health—good nutrition, regular exercise, keeping hydrated, sunlight and Vitamin D, avoiding things such as tobacco and alcohol, fresh air, proper rest and sleep, and an attitude of forgiveness and trust. And I wondered if there was one that I needed to focus on most. I had early morning classes, and I was working after school, so my life was pretty full. I noticed that when I went to bed late, the next day never went quite as well as it could have. Instead of getting up early and jogging for a mile, I would be tired and hit the snooze button several times. Instead of enjoying a healthful breakfast, I found myself looking for something a little sweeter, a little more processed—something to satisfy my feeling of "dis-ease." I just didn't feel as good as I did when I had gotten a good night's sleep the night before.

Have you experienced that? Do you make a habit of eating or drinking something first thing in the morning simply because you need it to "medicate" or improve the way you feel? I believe that millions of individuals in this world wake up in the morning with a sense of "dis-ease"—a sense that they just don't feel quite right. So they are looking for shortcuts to restore that feeling of wholeness, that feeling of wellness. Too often, those shortcuts are causing them to burn the candle at both ends, leading to adrenal fatigue and countless other physical and emotional problems.

I truly believe that sleep and proper rest is the most important key to regulating all the other health strategies, because if you are not waking up refreshed and restored, your body is not rejuvenating and healing itself during those hours of sleep as it is supposed to do.

> Sleep as a strategy for maximizing our healing potential includes so much more than most of us realize.

In today's fast-paced world, many of us feel we don't have time to get as much sleep as we need or as we would like. We are trying to fit everything in, and it just won't fit! So the hours for sleep are where we often make sacrifices. That thinking has destroyed generation after generation of people's health. Kids today are staying up until 1:00 and 2:00 o'clock in the morning, studying for exams or finishing school papers. They are destroying their health for the sake of a grade.

I would much rather my children get no A's at all in school and get a good night's sleep every night than for them to have a 4.0 GPA at the expense of their future health. Not getting enough sleep is setting up our children for all the chronic diseases that we are trying to prevent or reverse in adults. Sleep deprivation sets us up for obesity,[2] heart disease,[3] diabetes,[4] and Alzheimer's.[5] Loss of sleep is bad for physical, intellectual, and emotional health. It is especially bad for the brain.

THE NEGATIVE EFFECTS OF INADEQUATE SLEEP

One of my favorite stories when I was growing up was the story of Charles A. Lindberg, a dashing, young pilot in the days when flying was in its infancy.[6] In 1919 a New York City hotel owner offered a $25,000 prize to the first aviator to fly nonstop across the Atlantic Ocean from New York City to Paris. Lindbergh determined to be that aviator. He obtained financial backing and built a custom airplane, the *Spirit of St. Louis.* Although it was not a requirement for winning the prize, he decided to fly solo. This meant he would have to be at the controls for at least thirty hours. It actually turned out to be thirty-three hours.

On May 20, 1927, Lindberg took off from Roosevelt Field on Long Island. He was so excited that he didn't sleep at all the night before the flight. In fact, by the time he lifted off the ground, he had been without sleep for thirty hours. Lindberg became the first pilot to fly nonstop across the Atlantic, but oh how he wished many times during that thirty-three-hour flight to Paris that he had slept the night before!

He was fortunate to make it to Paris alive, very fortunate—and not just because of the limited aviation technology of that time. Sixty-three hours without sleep, even to accomplish such an amazing feat, exacts a tremendous toll on health and well-being

What does such sleep deprivation do to our genes? The Allen Institute for brain science reported that in studies on mice, some 224 genes showed a negatively changed genetic expression due to sleep deprivation and that thousands of genes appeared to be regulated by the 24-hour circadian rhythm.[7]

You might be thinking, *That's interesting. But that study involved mice, not human beings.* However, since that study, some great research in this area has been done on humans. One study, conducted by the University of Surrey in the United Kingdom and published in the *Proceedings of the National Academy of Sciences,* found that just one week of getting less than six hours of sleep each night significantly altered 711 genes, dramatically increasing inflammation.[8] We have seen repeatedly throughout this book how strongly inflammation is tied to disease. And one of the things that drives the body into an inflammatory state is inadequate sleep.

Even if you are exercising every day, even if you eating all the right foods, even if you are following all the other health strategies perfectly, if you are not getting enough sleep, that alone will increase inflammation. Sleep deprivation depresses immunity, causes stress to become chronic, and triggers metabolic problems.

Another study of young adults who went to bed at 3:00 in the morning, instead of at their usual bedtime, showed that the function of their immune system was depressed 50 percent.[9] The only variable in the study was the fact that they went to bed quite late. This means that the immune cells weren't doing their job destroying viruses and bacteria and other threats to their health. And all this is the result of only one night of poor sleep!

> Unfortunately, thousands of people wake up every morning with depressed immune cell activity due to not getting enough sleep. That alone could account for a significantly increased risk for all kinds of disease.

The study went on to show that after just one week of getting less than six hours of sleep a night, the cognitive thinking process was dramatically impaired.

DISRUPTING THE CIRCADIAN RHYTHM

Lest you think that it's only a matter of how much sleep one gets and that the timing isn't important, consider the results of another study conducted at the University of Surrey and published in 2014 in the *Proceedings of the National Academy of Science*.[10] In this study, researchers changed people's rhythm of sleep by moving sleep time from nighttime to the afternoon. Subjects in the study slept for six-and-half hours—from 12:00 noon until 6:30 P.M. What was the result?

Just three days of a disrupted sleep cycle significantly altered the expression of 1,172 of the 1,400 genes normally tied to the body's circadian rhythm. The researchers went on to suggest that sleep disruption ultimately affects about one-third of the entire human genome. That means that some 7,000 of the 20,000 genes in our body become dysfunctional simply because we are not sleeping according to the rhythm of nature.

Getting proper rest and enough sleep have critically important benefits for the body and for our health. We know, for example, that sleep helps neural functioning. We all know this intuitively. We know that when we get a good night's sleep and awake rested and refreshed, we have a different outlook on life than when we are not getting enough sleep. We can remember things better; our minds are clearer. We don't have that foggy, fuzzy feeling in our brain that I hear about so often from patients. Sleep gives our neurons a chance to recuperate.

CHILDREN AND ADEQUATE SLEEP

A study done by Dr. Eve Van Cauter[11] states that children under age 10 need about ten hours of sleep a day. This is an area in which society is really missing an opportunity to dramatically affect children's health in a positive way. Those between 12 and 21 years of age require about nine hours of sleep a day. Yet how many children and teenagers are getting adequate sleep? In this age group, sufficient sleep is important for brain development. It strengthens the immune system and contributes to good social behavior. British psychologist Tanya Byron has said, "Parents are ruining their children's lives by failing to teach them to sleep."[12]

> It's easy for us to blame a woman who is smoking or drinking during pregnancy for the way she is endangering the health and well-being of her unborn child. Yet how often do we think about what is happening to our children when we don't make sure they are getting adequate sleep, or when we aren't encouraging them to develop good sleep habits?

The International Journal of Obesity published a study in October 2010 showing that obesity rates increased for young children who had less than seven or eight hours of sleep a night. For boys 4 to 8 years old, there was a 300 percent increase. For girls 9 to 13 years old, the increase in obesity rates was 500 percent.[13]

How could just this one factor—inadequate sleep—have such a huge impact on obesity in children? We usually think of obesity as a problem caused by overeating or lack of exercise. And, of course, those things are certainly part of the problem. But we need to be looking at the bigger picture and ask, "What are the factors that cause a person to choose to eat a cookie or a bag of chips, instead of a piece of fruit?

BURNING THE MIDNIGHT OIL

If you were in the military, you probably heard one of your superior officers warn you as you were being released for week-end leave, "Nothing good happens after midnight. Be in bed before midnight." If you played college athletics of any kind, your coach probably told you the same thing. "Be in bed before midnight; nothing good happens after that." But the value of that advice goes far beyond just the notion of avoiding bad situations that are likely to get you into trouble. This is also good advice for health and for other aspects of life.

When it comes to academic performance, for example, if you choose to burn the midnight oil in order to gain more knowledge, or do well on a test, or finish an assignment, you are going against what science is telling us about rest, brain activity, and mental efficiency.

> When you have a lot to do, when you're feeling overwhelmed, when you're trying to fix information in your mind, the scientific evidence indicates that the best strategy is to get plenty of rest before tackling the task at hand.

I've watched individuals who were facing hard classes or important exams, and I've noticed something interesting. The night before a test, for example, some would go to bed at 9:00 P.M. and sleep until 3:00 A.M., at which time they would wake up and begin studying. Others would study until midnight and sleep until 6:00 A.M. Both were getting the same amount of sleep—six hours. But those who went to sleep early before getting up to study did better. Even though they were getting only six hours of sleep, going to bed at 9:00 P.M. greatly enhanced the quality of that sleep and increased its potential to restore the brain and body. Studies have shown that getting to bed at a reasonable hour is a strong predictor of GPA in college.[14]

In 2014, Drs. Roxane Prichard and Monica Hartmann, both professors at University of St. Thomas, analyzed data from 43,000 college students across the United States and discovered that sleep timing and sleep-related problems were far more related to poor academic performance than were binge drinking, marijuana use, and even illicit drug use![15] Of course, based on what we are discussing in this chapter, consistently going to sleep at least one or two hours before midnight would likely make it a lot easier to avoid alcohol and drugs. Good sleep habits make us feel much better and make us less likely to start looking for unhealthy shortcuts that temporarily boost or calm our mood.

STAYING TRUE TO YOUR BIOLOGICAL CLOCK

If you aren't consistently getting a good night's sleep, a new study suggests you could be reducing your ability to lower oxidative stress.[16] Uncontrolled oxidation is one of the primary toxins that leads to heart disease, promotes cancer, and causes strokes, autoimmune problems, and inflammation. It accelerates aging and increases motor and neurological deterioration.

A good night's sleep may be one of the most important antioxidants available to us, preventing the oxidation from occurring in the first place.

While discussing his 2010 study published in the journal, *Aging*, Dr. Krishnan, a professor at Oregon State University, stated that young people ". . . may be able to handle certain stresses, but the same . . . [stresses] at an older age cause genetic damage and appear to lead to health problems and earlier death. And it's linked to biological clocks."[17] These studies demonstrate that inadequate sleep, or simply going to bed late, will disrupt the way our circadian clock genes function. If the circadian clock gene is expressed in unhealthy ways and damaged, it will greatly reduce our ability to handle the toxic effects of oxidative stress on our health.

Our bodies are very resilient and appear to handle significant abuse when we are young, but these unhealthy behaviors in our teens and early twenties alter the function of our genes, leading to premature aging and dysfunction. A large study of 70,000 women conducted by Harvard University found that those who slept five hours a night had a 40 percent higher rate of heart attacks than did those who slept eight hours.[18] We need to be true to our biological clocks.

When the International Agency for Research on Cancer ranked various causes of cancer in 2009, it placed working the night shift just below exposure to known carcinogens, such as asbestos, as a cause of cancer.[19] Our biological clocks play a much greater role in our health than we realize. The human body seems designed to be active during daylight hours and to use the hours of darkness for rest and rejuvenation. When we disrupt that cycle for any reason, we disrupt the body's ability to optimize health. We put a great deal of emphasis on toxins from our environment, as we should. But it is also critically important to understand that appropriate sleep is one of the most important strategies for removing toxins from the brain. More on this later in this chapter.

SLEEP AND INSULIN RESISTANCE

Not getting enough sleep leads to hepatic and peripheral insulin resistance. In non-medical jargon, that means that when you don't sleep well or you don't sleep enough, your liver becomes very resistant to insulin.[20] As a result, it starts dumping sugar into the bloodstream. This is one reason so many people with prediabetes or diabetes have high blood sugars first thing in the morning—often much higher than they do after they eat. When the liver becomes resistant to insulin, the pancreas compensates by producing a tremendous amount of insulin. It is trying to force the liver to reabsorb some of that sugar. But the liver isn't the only place insulin resistance can develop; it also happens in the muscles.

When the muscles become resistant to insulin, blood sugars shoot up, causing the pancreas to produce even more insulin. Since elevated insulin promotes fat storage, this process is one of the main factors driving obesity.

Think of all the different hormones in your body as participants in a symphony. For this symphony to make beautiful music, each hormone must play its part and be in sync with the others. What would happen in an orchestra if the violins or the horns just started going their own way with no regard for the other instruments? It would ruin the experience of the symphony. That is something like what happens when insulin levels become erratic. Insulin is one of the most dominant hormones in the body. When insulin levels become excessive and dysfunctional, they negatively influence cortisol balance. Fluctuation of the stress hormone, cortisol, will lead to many undesirable health effects and symptoms, including fluctuation of many other hormones. This can lead to a "roller coaster" effect on levels of energy, our mood, ability to concentrate, and can greatly influence our ability to make good decisions. There are long-term effects as well. Insulin resistance, with its resulting excess insulin production, is the primary factor promoting cardiovascular disease.[21] And it is a major factor in such common cancers as breast,[22] prostate,[23] and colon[24] cancers.

SLEEP AND MELATONIN PRODUCTION

At a meeting of the American Association of Cancer Researchers in early 2014, researcher Sarah Mark reported on a study showing that men with high levels of melatonin had a 75 percent lower risk of developing advanced prostate cancer. They also had better insulin control.[25]

How does the body produce more melatonin? Interestingly, it depends on being in sync with your body's circadian rhythm, the body's biological clock. The first thing that determines whether your pineal gland is able to release a high level of melatonin at night, when it is dark, is whether you have spent some time in the sunlight during the previous day. This is a key determinant of how well your body heals and restores its body functions while you sleep.

Early morning, when the sun is just coming up, is the best time to get outside in the bright light. Your goal should be to spend at least a half-hour in bright light every day, preferably in the morning.

When you are in the sunlight, the photons in that light go right through the eye and are transmitted by the optic nerve to the brain center that regulates the circadian clock genes. This, in turn, resets the pineal gland, increasing its ability to release melatonin when it's dark and you are asleep. If you have spent enough time in the sunlight, the pineal gland is able to release a much higher amount of melatonin at night, but only if the lights are out and it is dark.[26] Getting morning sunlight and going to bed by 10:00 P.M. will likely optimize your body's ability to produce melatonin and maximize your healing potential.

You see, your body's ability to release melatonin depends on timing and your circadian rhythm. Timing is everything when it comes to the processes that affect your health. The timing of when you sleep, when you wake up, when you eat—are all part of your circadian rhythm and have a powerful influence on your health and healing potential. Timing, therefore, can either optimize or minimize the potential benefits of a particular activity.

INADEQUATE SLEEP AND OBESITY

A study published in the *Journal of Clinical Endocrinology and Metabolism* in 2010 showed that people who were getting only five to six hours of sleep a night had a 69 percent greater risk for obesity, compared to those getting seven to eight hours. The effect of inadequate sleep is also determined by how long we persist in poor sleep habits. A study done in Spain showed that lack of sleep strongly promoted weight gain over time.

Compared to women who slept seven hours each night, women getting less than five hours of sleep were over three times more likely to gain twelve pounds during the next two years.[27] That's six extra pounds per year of poor sleep habits.

Some people don't become too concerned about increased risk factors for various diseases, but they are concerned about their appearance. Of course, obesity affects both our health *and* our appearance. I believe we should be very much involved in our health and do everything we can to be as healthy as possible. But I also understand the importance of appearance.

We all want to put our best foot forward, to look as good as possible. So that is yet another factor to think about in connection with getting enough sleep.

There is little doubt that poor sleep habits negatively affect our appearance. The only proof we need is to stay up late and then look in the mirror the next morning.

INSOMNIA

Insomnia is often stress-induced, and it doesn't have to be extreme stress or something obvious that is visibly affecting our lives. There is so much stress in our world as a matter of course that insomnia can be caused by just the chronic, repetitive, low-grade stress that comes from living in today's world.

Stress causes the adrenal glands to release cortisol. There is a certain level of cortisol that the body needs. But when we are under chronic stress, the adrenal glands are perpetually producing too much cortisol.

That can continue only so long; the body can't continue to produce high levels of cortisol indefinitely. After years or decades of poorly managed stress, the adrenals eventually become worn out, and adrenal fatigue sets in.

INSOMNIA AND ADRENAL FATIGUE

Many individuals who have been living active lives, operating for years under chronic stress and producing a lot of cortisol, find as they reach middle age, that their body isn't able to handle that any longer. The body starts producing less cortisol, blood sugars drop, and that is when they often start experiencing unusual cravings. They begin wanting to eat things they know are not good for them. They become unwilling to do things they know they should do in order to have good health. A common example is no longer putting effort toward getting daily exercise. They simply stop making good decisions about their health.

They often begin to feel fatigued mid-to-late morning and especially mid-to-late afternoon. This is because their cortisol levels are fluctuating unhealthfully throughout the day—up too much and then down too much, back and forth. Because the fatigued adrenals are not able to maintain a steady level of cortisol production, they under-produce cortisol for several hours, followed by over-production when the blood sugars become too low. This is the hallmark of "adrenal fatigue" which influences every aspect of our health.[28]

But for many individuals in this group, the energy comes back around 7:00 or 8:00 P.M. They begin feeling good again. By 9:00 o'clock they are feeling *really* good, and getting ready for bed is the last thing on their mind. They should be preparing to be in bed by 10:00 so they can start producing melatonin and begin repairing their body and brain for the demands of the next day. But they are feeling great! At 9:30, 10:00, even 11:00 o'clock, they are going strong. *I've felt tired all day,* they tell themselves. *I just want to stay up and feel good a little longer.* That's understandable. But the problem is that they are sacrificing tomorrow's energy in order to feel good right now.

Dealing with this is a challenge, because if you find yourself in this situation, it really is difficult for you to go to sleep at this point. The level of cortisol and other stress hormones in your body is not back up to a level that would be healthy if it were morning. But it's night-time. All the body systems are activated and ready to go.

> The solution involves stepping back and reestablishing the various health strategies, reincorporating them into your life, and letting them calm the mind and relax the body for sleep at a reasonable time.

Getting outside in the early morning is one of the first strategies to address in combating adrenal fatigue and insomnia. If you're not sleeping well, the tendency is to sleep in when morning comes. That is one of the most common mistakes made by people who have insomnia. You need to get up at a reasonable time so that you can get outside and experience thirty minutes of bright-light therapy. That's critical for breaking the dysrhythmia that you are caught in. You have to break that cycle first thing in the morning with bright light.[29]

Next, try to take advantage of some exercise along with the early morning sunshine. It doesn't need to be vigorous; walking is fine. Try to get some additional moderate exercise during the day. Your exercise should be moderate, but enough to cause you to sweat. Sweating will not only help detoxify your body, it will also help calm you physically, which in turn calms the mind. An overactive mind is frequently associated with an under-exercised body.

PROGRESSIVE MUSCLE RELAXATION

Another strategy I recommend to individuals struggling with insomnia is progressive muscle relaxation. If you're finding it difficult to fall asleep at night and you're feeling tense and anxious, try some progressive muscle relaxation. Start by making a fist with both hands. For six seconds, make a fist just as tight and hard as you can. Then take a deep breath, release the fist, and as you release that deep breath, concentrate on feeling the stress leaving your fingertips. Feel the relaxation and the release of tension in those muscles.

Then you just progressively move up, muscle group after muscle group. Next, do the same with the forearm; tense the forearm for six seconds and then concentrate on letting all that tension drain away. Continue with the biceps and shoulders, the neck, the face, the back muscles, the chest muscles—work all the way down the body and end with your toes. It is very therapeutic, and it's something you can do anywhere. This is an excellent way to rid yourself of tension and restore your body's rhythms.

INSOMNIA AND EATING BEFORE BEDTIME

Another key strategy in combating insomnia is not eating late.[30] That can be difficult. Whenever we're feeling depressed and anxious or happy and excited, one of the first impulses that comes to mind is, *Hey! I know how to make this better. I'm going to eat something!*

Whether things are really bad or really good, we want to eat something.

However, research tells us that to optimize the benefits of sleep, it's best to have about three to four hours between the evening meal and the time we go to bed.[31] This is especially important if you are one of those individuals who aren't able to fall asleep easily around 10:00 or 10:30 P.M.

Chronic adrenal fatigue that causes the blood sugars to drop significantly during the night can be one of the main causes of night-time wakefulness. Some people are able to fall asleep at 10:00 o'clock without much difficulty, but by 2:00 or 3:00 A.M. they are wide awake. They haven't had enough sleep, and they certainly have not had enough restorative sleep, the kind that research shows is necessary for detoxifying the body—regenerating and rejuvenating it.

One of the more common reasons for this abrupt, 2:00 A.M. wake-up call is blood sugars that have dipped too low. When the blood sugars reach a certain low point, alarms will go off in the brain alerting it to the problem. These alarms tell the adrenal glands to release the stress hormone, cortisol.[32] In response, the liver begins to release its sugar stores to bring the blood sugar levels back up to normal. By this time, you have stress hormones surging through your blood. These stress hormones are supposed to be released and increased gradually over the hours before you wake up. Cortisol should act like a dimmer switch, the level slowly rising until 9:00 A.M. so that when you wake up and begin your day's activities you feel refreshed and energetic.[33] The idea is to keep you from waking up suddenly, startled out of a sound sleep. Adrenal fatigue is very closely associated with inadequate and poor-quality sleep. So it's important to correct it.

SLEEP DEPRIVATION AND MOTOR SKILLS

Several studies have shown that sleep deprivation can impair your judgment and motor skills even more than alcohol intoxication does.[34] One such study involved young mothers with small children. These young women were not getting enough sleep because of having to care for infants, and the quality of the sleep they did get was poor. When these sleep-deprived moms were placed in auto driving simulators and asked to negotiate various traffic routes, they made 30 percent more driving mistakes and misjudgments than did a control group of young mothers who were intoxicated from drinking alcohol!

Fatigue impairs judgment and reaction time as much or more than does exposure to alcohol.[35] Studies in Oklahoma and California showed that 50 percent of fatal accidents on freeways are due to sleep problems.

THE BIOLOGICAL CLOCK IN YOUR BRAIN

Let's go back to the biological clock in your brain. Human beings have an internal biological clock that is synchronized with the cycle of light and dark, day and night, in the physical world. Have you ever seen someone who is really burned out, who just can't handle life as they used to be able to? New studies are showing that burnout is directly related to the ability of sleep to rejuvenate and restore the brain to optimal function.

In October, 2013, Dr. Maiken Nedergaard, at the University of Rochester, published a study in the *Journal of Science* that caught my attention. In it, he states that the byproducts of day-time brain function must be detoxified at night. This is accomplished by the glymphatic system pumping cerebral spinal fluid through the brain at night, flushing toxins into the circulation and to the liver.[36]

This is a new concept. The byproducts of day-time brain function must be detoxified at night. Did you ever think that your brain is actually generating toxins all day long as a byproduct of what it is doing? We have to deal with those toxins somehow; they cannot stay in the brain, or it will become neurotoxic.

> We know from metabolic research that the brain is one of the most metabolically active organs in the body. A significant percentage of the carbohydrates that we consume in a given day will be used by the brain.[37]

"Seventy-five percent of the energy derived and stored by the body from carbohydrates is ultimately used by the body to sustain brain function."[38] We have a hard time visualizing that, because we think of the brain as just sitting there, not doing any physical work. Actually, it is working tremendously hard, and that means it is naturally producing toxins that will need to be flushed out of the system.

The brain has its own detoxifying system that washes and flushes itself out every night. It's something like washing out a paint brush after use, so that it will be ready to be used the next day. The brain does the same thing at night. But why does the glymphatic brain detoxification system work mainly at night?

Some have compared this nightly cleansing of the brain to having a party at your house. While the party is going on and there are people everywhere enjoying a good meal and social activity—that is not the time to clean the house. You clean after the party is over and everyone has gone home. Your brain can't function and clean itself up at the same time. Detoxifying the brain is such an important task that it takes place at night while we're fast asleep. That's when the glymphatic system cleans toxins from the brain. Isn't that amazing? Our bodies and our brains are fearfully and wonderfully made. But we have to give them time to heal every night. And if we don't give them proper rest, we're extending the amount of time our brains are exposed to toxins.

There is speculation by some scientists that one reason Alzheimer's is increasing exponentially in our society is because we're not giving the brain adequate time to detoxify at night. It's important that we allow the biological clock in our brain to cleanse itself and reset itself every night. That is yet another reason a good night's sleep is so vitally important.

OPTIMIZING SLEEP FOR MAXIMUM WELL-BEING

We were designed for joy and health. But we're not going to experience that unless we take advantage of restorative sleep. Nothing tends to promote health of body and spirit more than an attitude of praise and gratitude. But we're not going to be able to have that kind of attitude unless we clear our brains of toxins each night through restorative sleep. You can enjoy each day in a way that gives you even more joy tomorrow, but only if you optimize the benefits of a good night's sleep.

CHAPTER SUMMARY

>> Adequate sleep is the most important key to regulating all the other health strategies.

>> Without adequate sleep, your body is unable to rejuvenate itself as it is supposed to.

>> Children under age 10 need about ten hours of sleep a day. Those between 12 and 21 years of age require about nine hours of sleep a day.

>> College coaches often tell their athletes, "Nothing good happens after midnight. Be in bed before midnight."

>> Going to bed late and having sleep-related problems are far more related to poor academic performance than are binge drinking, marijuana use, and even illicit drug use!

>> Inadequate sleep drives the body into an inflammatory state, making it susceptible to disease.

>> Not only the amount of sleep, but the timing of sleep is important. Disrupting sleep and the circadian rhythm alters the genetic expression of over 7,000 genes. That's one-third of our entire genome.

>> Working the night shift is listed just below exposure to known carcinogens as a cause of cancer.

>> The human body seems designed to be active during daylight hours and to use the hours of darkness for rest and rejuvenation.

>> Compared to women who sleep seven hours each night, women getting less than five hours of sleep are more than three times more likely to gain one pound every two months.

>> Years of unhealthy sleep habits promote both prediabetes and reactive hypoglycemia, often resulting in adrenal fatigue.

>> Getting outside in the early morning for exercise and sunlight exposure is a key strategy in combating adrenal fatigue and insomnia.

>> To optimize the benefits of sleep, it's best to have about three to four hours between the evening meal and the time we go to bed.

>> The glymphatic system is the brain's personal detoxifier, pumping cerebral spinal fluid through the brain at night and flushing toxins into the circulatory system.

ENDNOTES

1 White, Ellen G., *The Ministry of Healing* (Mountain View, CA: Pacific Press, 1905).

2 de Jong, E.; et al., "Association Between Sleep Duration and Overweight: The Importance of Parenting," *International Journal of Obesity*, (2012) 36, 1278–1284; doi:10.1038/ijo.2012.119; published online July 24, 2012.

3 Patel, Sanjay; White, David P.; Buysse, Daniel J.; Blaivas, Allen, "Sleep and Heart Disease: What's the Link?" Video transcript. http://sciencedaily.healthology.com/sleep-disorders/sleep-disorders-information/video2940.htm.

4 Donga, E., "A Single Night of Partial Sleep Deprivation Induces Insulin Resistance in Multiple Metabolic Pathways in Healthy Subjects," *Journal of Clinical Endocrinology and Metabolism,* June 2010; 95(6): 2963-2968. doi: 10.1210/jc.2009-2430.

5 Spira, Adam P., et al., "Self-Reported Sleep and ß-Amyloid Deposition in Community-Dwelling Older Adults," *Journal of the American Medical Association Neurology*, October 21, 2013; doi:10.1001/jamaneurol.2013.4258.

6 Lindbergh, Charles A., *The Spirit of St. Louis* (New York, NY: Avon, 1953).

7 Allen Institute for Brain Science and SRI International, November 2007, http://help.brain-map.org/display/mousebrain/Documentation.

8 Möller-Levet, Carla S., et al., "Effects of Insufficient Sleep on Circadian Rhythmicity and Expression Amplitude of the Human Blood Transcriptome," *PNAS Plus - Biological Sciences - Medical Sciences*, PNAS (2013) 110 (12) E1132-E1141; published ahead of print February 25, 2013, doi:10.1073/pnas.1217154110.

9 Michael, Irwin, et al., "Partial Night Sleep Deprivation Reduces Natural Killer and Cellular Immune Responses in Humans," *Federation of American Societies for Experimental Biology Journal*, 10 (1996):643-653.

10 Archer, Simon N., et al., "Mistimed Sleep Disrupts Circadian Regulation of the Human Transcriptome," *PNAS Plus - Biological Sciences - Medical Sciences:* PNAS 2014 111 (6) E682-E691; published ahead of print January 21, 2014, doi:10.1073/pnas.1316335111.

11 Dr. Eve Van Cauter's works include Spiegel, K.; Leproult, R.; Van Cauter, E., "Impact of a Sleep Debt on Metabolic and Endocrine Function," *The Lancet,* 354 (1999): 1435-1439, and Spiegel, K.; Leproult, R.; L'Hermite-Balériaux, R.; Copinschi, G.; Penev, P.; Van Cauter, E., "Impact of Sleep Duration on the 24-Hour Leptin Profile: Relationships with Sympatho-Vagal Balance, Cortisol and TSH," *Journal of Clinical Endocrinology and Metabolism,* 89, No. 11 (November 2004) 5762-5771.

12 http://www.telegraph.co.uk/news/health/children/9923378/Parents-ruining-childrens-lives-by-failing-to-teach-them-to-sleep-Tanya-Byron-says.html

13 de Jong, E., et al., "Association Between Sleep Duration and Overweight: The Importance of Parenting," *International Journal of Obesity,* (2012) 36, 1278-1284; doi:10.1038/ijo.2012.119; published online July 24, 2012.

14 Lowry, M., et al., "The Link Between Sleep Quantity and Academic Performance for the College Student," *Sentience: The University of Minnesota Undergraduate Journal of Psychology*, Vol. 3, Spring 2010.

15 Prichard, J.; Hartmann, M., "What is the Cost of Poor Sleep for College Students Calculating the Contribution of Academic Sleep Failures Using a Large National Sample," *Journal of Sleep and Sleep Disorders Research*, 28th Annual Meeting of the Associated Professional Sleep Societies, Vol. 37, Abstract Supplement 1068 (2012).

16 Krishnan, N.; Kretzschmar, D.; Rakshit, K.; Chow, E.; Giebultowicz, J., "The Circadian Clock Gene Period Extends Healthspan in Aging Drosophila Melanogaster," *Aging.* (2009) 1:937-948.

17 http://phys.org/news186683062.html

18 Patel, Sanjay; White, David P.; Buysse, Daniel J.; Blaivas, Allen, "Sleep and Heart Disease: What's the Link?" Video transcript. http://sciencedaily.healthology.com/sleep-disorders/sleep-disorders-information/video2940.htm.

19 MacDonald, Kenneth, "Night Shifts Spark Cancer Pay-out," BBC News online, March 15, 2009. http://news.bbc.co.uk/2/hi/uk_news/scotland/7945145.stm.

20 Donga, E., "A Single Night of Partial Sleep Deprivation Induces Insulin Resistance in Multiple Metabolic Pathways in Healthy Subjects," *Journal of Clinical Endocrinology and Metabolism,* June 2010; 95(6):2963-2968. doi: 10.1210/jc.2009-2430.

21 Eddy, D., "Relationship of Insulin Resistance and Related Metabolic Variables to Coronary Artery Disease: A Mathematical Analysis," *Diabetes Care,* 32 (2009), 361-366.

22 Novosyadly, Ruslan; LeRoith, Derek, "Hyperinsulinemia and Type 2 Diabetes," *Cell Cycle,* 9.8 (2010), 1449, 1450.

23 James, Barnard, R., "Prostate Cancer Prevention by Nutritional Means to Alleviate Metabolic Syndrome," *The American Journal of Clinical Nutrition,* 86.3 (2007), 8895-8935.

24 Giovannucci, Edward, "Insulin and Colon Cancer," *Cancer Causes and Control,* 6.2 (1995), 164-179.

25 American Association for Cancer Research (AACR), "Melatonin May Lower Prostate Cancer Risk," *Science Daily,* (January 20, 2014). Retrieved April 10, 2015 from www.sciencedaily.com/releases/2014/01/140120085058.htm

26 Laakso, M., et al, "Twenty-Four Hour Patters of Pineal Melatonin and Pituitary and Plasma Prolactin in Male Rats Under 'Natural' and Artificial Lighting Conditions," *Neuroendocrinology,* September 1988; 48(3): 308-313.

27 López-García, E., et al., "Sleep Duration, General and Abdominal Obesity and Weight Change Among the Older Adult Population of Spain," *American Journal of Clinical Nutrition,* February 2008; 87(2): 310-316.

28 Wilson, James, "Adrenal Fatigue: The 21st Century Stress Syndrome," (Smart Publications, 2002).

29 Wagner, D., "Sleep Disorders: Disorders of the Circadian Sleep-Wake Cycle," *Neurologic Clinics,* August 1996; 14(3); 651.

30 Afaghi, A., et al., "High-Glycemic-Index Carbohydrate Meals Shorten Sleep Onset," *American Journal of Clinical Nutrition,* February 2007; 85: 2 426-430.

31 Dollander, M., "Etiology of Adult Insomnia," *Encephale,* (2002) 28:493-502.

32 Rodenbeck, A., "Interactions Between Evening and Nocturnal Cortisol Secretion and Sleep Parameters in Patients with Seere 41 Chronic Primary Insomnia," *Neuroscience Letters,* (2002) 324:159-163.

33 Balbo, M., "Impact of Sleep and Its Disturbances on Hypothalamo-Pituitary-Adrenal Axis Activity," *International Journal of Endocrinology,* (2010) Article ID 759234, 16 pages. doi:10.1155/2010/759234.

34 Haraldsson, P., et al., "Drowsiness—Greater Traffic Hazard Than Alcohol. Causes, Risks and Treatment," *Lakartidningen,* 98, No. 25 (June 20, 2001) 3018-3023.

35 Arnedt, J. T., et al., "How Do Prolonged Wakefulness and Alcohol Compare in the Decrements They Produce on a Simulated Driving Task?" *Accident Analysis & Prevention,* (2001) 33:337-344.

36 Xie, L.; Nedergaard, M., "Sleep Drives Metabolite Clearance from the Adult Brain," *Science,* October 18, 2013; 342 (6156), 373-377. DOI:10.1126/science.1241224.

37 http://www.livescience.com/3186-brain-food-eat-smart.html

38 http://www.faqs.org/sports-science/Ba-Ca/Carbohydrate-Stores-Muscle-Glycogen-Liver-Glycogen-and-Glucose.html

— T W E L V E —

Testing... Testing...

CHOOSING THE BEST
CLINICAL LAB TESTS

A FEW MONTHS AGO, ANN CAME TO SEE ME. SHE HAD
noticed a lump in her armpit while taking a shower. Thinking this might well
be cancer and being very afraid of conventional therapies, she came to me.
She was worried and upset. She didn't want to face the possibilities; she didn't
want to go there at all.

I knew what my primary job was in this situation. My job would be to
help Ann determine and become aware of what was really going on and to
embrace the reality. To that end, one of the first things I did was to tell her the
story of Norman Cousins. You see, I knew that when we start avoiding what
might be, we often miss opportunities to find healing.

Norman Cousins, political journalist, author, and professor, was diagnosed
with a terminal illness—a lethal form of ankylosing spondylitis, at that time
known as Marie-Strumpell's disease. He said to the physician, "What are my
chances?"

The young doctor looked at him and said, "Well, it's terminal. You need to
get your life in order."

Cousins repeated, "Doctor, I want to know what my chances are."

The specialist once again tried to explain to Mr. Cousins that he had an incurable condition. Finally Cousins was able to make him understand that he wanted to know if anyone survived this disease. The physician went to the medical library and found a study showing that only one person out of 500 survived that diagnosis. He went to Cousin's hospital room to deliver the bad news.

Cousins responded, "One out of 500! I'm going to be that one!"

"No! No!" the doctor tried to calm him down. "You need to stay here and take the medication and treatment we recommend."

"Why would I want to stay in a place where I'm being told I'm going to die?" Cousins demanded.

EMBRACING THE DIAGNOSIS

The point of the story is that Norman Cousins embraced the diagnosis, but he denied and defied the verdict that it was inevitably terminal. One of the most significant components of optimizing your health, your potential for healing, is to embrace the diagnosis. Find out what's wrong. Find out what is missing that is necessary for health. And when you do that, it can lead, in some very unexpected ways, to healing.

Norman Cousins went on to write a book about his experience, *The Anatomy of an Illness*. It contains some extremely insightful statements:

"Each patient carries his own doctor inside him."

"I have learned never to underestimate the capacity of the human mind and body to regenerate—even when prospects seem most wretched. The life force may be the least understood force on earth."

"The control center of your life is your attitude."

After receiving the diagnosis of a terminal illness, Cousins determined to do anything possible to defy the odds. His research assistant at the *Saturday Review* began to work the phones trying to find anything that might help his boss. After an exhaustive review of every possible lead, he came up with only two things—megadoses of Vitamin C taken intravenously and a positive attitude of faith, hope, and laughter. Of course, these were long shots, but what did Cousins have to lose? He would work with what he had.

"I made the joyous discovery," he wrote, "that ten minutes of genuine belly laughter had an anesthetic effect and would give me at least two hours of pain-free sleep." This aspect of his treatment—laughter and a positive attitude—we know today as "active stress."

> Passive stress is a debilitating resignation to the harmful, negative things that come to us. Active stress, on the other hand, is a reaction that resolves to meet these stresses of life with a positive, optimistic attitude.

Active stress has a significantly beneficial effect on the immune system. King Solomon prophetically encapsulated this principle in these words: "A merry heart does good, like a medicine, but a broken spirit dries the bones."[1]

I shared this story with Ann, but I could tell that she wasn't fully convinced. She had been told she should have a CT scan. She didn't want to do that, because she was afraid of what it would reveal. She had been doing some research and suspected she had some kind of breast cancer or perhaps Non-Hodgkin's Lymphoma. She didn't want to know. She didn't want to hear her options.

I suggested she should have the CT scan. "Find out what's going on," I urged. "And in the meantime, let's do a comprehensive evaluation of your health. Let's find out what you can start fixing right now—things that are interrelated with whatever you're most concerned about."

It took a little encouragement, but a few weeks later she had completed a whole series of tests. The CT scan showed everything was basically normal. The lump under her arm turned out to be a lipoma, an abnormal fat growth that was totally benign. That happens sometimes. You can get them on your back, arms, or legs, and they can appear other places on the body. They are nothing to worry about. They can be easily removed surgically. But sometimes they really scare people. That benign lipoma gave Ann an opportunity to step back and evaluate her health in a comprehensive way.

INITIATING AN EFFECTIVE WELLNESS PROGRAM

What is the best way to initiate an effective wellness program and motivate yourself to follow it? We've looked at various strategies for health throughout this book, but how do we actually find the motivation to initiate and maintain an effective wellness program?

In Chapter 3, I mentioned that when I was in my 20s I thought I was Mr. Fitness. I was young and fit; I thought I was really healthy. But I'd never taken the time to actually evaluate my internal health. I'd done all kinds of tests to evaluate my physical fitness. I worked hard on a regular basis to be above the 90th percentile in every fitness category. All through college I worked hard at being fit, and I assumed that being fit meant that I was healthy.

Then one fateful day at the age of 24 I took a free cholesterol screening test and discovered that there was an inconsistency between my view of my health and what my body actually showed as a result of medical testing. My cholesterol was 244—well above the 95th percentile for my age. Not only was it high, it was off the chart—literally. The graph on the report didn't have a place to put that number. Believe me, that experience motivated me to start a solid wellness program!

> For all of us, the goal is to maximize our healing potential. We may be feeling great now, but we also want to optimize our potential for health and wellness into the future.

How can we best do this? What are the best lab tests to help us know exactly where we stand healthwise—so we can plan how best to optimize our wellbeing?

Over two thousand years ago, at the height of Roman rule over the world, an individual named Jesus came on the stage of human history. We still use his birth to date events as occurring "B.C." or "A.D." When he spoke, Jesus often attracted large crowds, because for the first time in many years people saw someone who was speaking truth with authority. They were thirsty for this kind of teaching. On one occasion, Jesus turned to those who were following him and said, "Suppose one of you wants to build a tower. Wouldn't you first sit down and estimate the cost to see if you have enough money to complete it?"[2] He loved causing people to think things through carefully. Years before Jesus' time on earth, there was a Jewish proverb that echoed a similar thought: "Plans fail for lack of counsel, but with many advisors they succeed." I'd like to suggest that when we fail at a wellness program, it's because we're not planning properly.

It's easy to plan improperly as we begin a wellness program—or not to plan at all. If you don't have a sense of what's really going on in your body or what your health problems might be, you may just start following some wellness strategies and do this or that, without thinking it all through as a whole. How can a person stay motivated in a program without knowing his or her baseline assessment? That's one of the most fundamental, and most important, things to know.

If you truly want to optimize your health, you have to be willing, like Norman Cousins, to embrace the diagnosis. That means being willing to find out what is actually going on in your body, and that requires testing.

So let's not ignore the diagnostics. Let's find out what's going on and accept reality. Then we can defy the verdict!

That's the exciting part. That's the part I love being involved in—defying the verdict, reversing disease where possible, helping people optimize their health.

The first step in properly understanding and then treating the main causes of disease is assessment. You need to ask, "Where are the gaps in my journey of wellness? Where are the potholes that can trip me up and create barriers to healing unless they are discovered and addressed directly?"

I believe that science now has the knowledge and the tools to provide profound, personalized healthcare if we take advantage of comprehensive testing. This includes genetic testing. We're at a stage of scientific knowledge regarding the human genome that allows us to learn a great deal about our genes—how they work and what the problem is when they don't work as they should.

One example is the aging process. As we get older, we discover that we're not as agile or strong as we once were. It takes longer to come up with names and information than it did when we were younger. Is this inevitable? Must we accept this as just a natural part of aging? Or is something else happening as we age that is contributing to this slowing down?

Can we modify the aging process or even control it based on a better understanding of our unique, genetic self?

Genetic testing can help us answer those questions. The Roman philosopher, Cicero, wrote, "Old age must be resisted and its deficiencies supplied."

There are some 20,000 genes in the human genome. Among these 20,000 genes are many genetic mutations. We all have them; they are just different for each of us. By understanding where these mutation occur and by recognizing the biochemical pathways in the body that are well-established, we can determine exactly which nutrients relate to that enzymatic pathway that is not working optimally because of a particular genetic mutation. This gives us a lot of additional control over our genes that we didn't have previously. So dysfunctional genes must be detected, then supported holistically, and finally nutrigenomically bypassed in order to supply their associated nutrient deficiencies. This is the exciting field of genetic engineering by the appropriate use of nutritional principles.

Some scientists consider the finding of the methyltetrahydofolate reductase gene, called MTHFR, to be the most exciting genetic discovery since the human genome project was completed in 2003. This gene, when mutated significantly, decreases your potential to heal damaged DNA, detoxify old hormones, and prevent viruses from replicating. If one parent has passed on to you a normal copy of this MTHFR gene, but the other parent has given you a mutated copy, your body's ability to activate folate has been diminished by about 40 percent. If you have received a mutated copy of this gene from both parents, this dysfunction increases up to 70 percent.[3][4] This has the potential to have a profound effect on your health. But the good news is that we now know exactly how to bypass the effect of that gene mutation. Specifically, we know how to bypass the negative effects of this mutation using the appropriate nutrients. That's the kind of knowledge we are gaining from the study of the human genome. And that points out the importance of genetic testing.

My patients are strongly encouraged to take advantage of genetic testing. Even though genetic testing is not typically covered by health insurance, there are affordable options. At www.23andme.com a simple saliva sample can provide information on hundreds of genes for only $99. You can order it yourself. Within three to five weeks you will receive an email explaining how to access the data file on your genes. Then you can use www.geneticgenie.org and www.mthfrsupport.com to generate reports detailing which genes are normal and whether some have one or two mutated copies. Of course, as with any form of lab testing, you will want to work with a medical professional who is knowledgeable in the clinical applications of genetic testing. That could include your family physician, a lifestyle medicine doctor, a clinical nutritionist, or functional medicine specialist. When reviewing genetic testing it is always important to compare the results with those of all your other lab tests as well as with your personal medical history. Done properly, this takes one or more sixty-minute consultations.

> A critical principle in gene testing is that one gene does not make a person. Having one mutated gene or one normal gene doesn't determine who you are.

After all, we have 20,000 genes in our genome, so it's the inter-relationship between all these genes and how they are expressed or deactivated epigenetically that ultimately determines health or disease.

THE ARCHIMEDES STUDY

In Chapter 1 we looked at the Archimedes Study conducted by Dr. David Eddy.[5] That study was seeking to determine which risk factors have the most impact on whether an individual develops heart disease. And, as we saw in Chapter 1, the study found that family history accounts for only about 4 percent of the risk of having heart disease.

Family history is important. It's part of the initial assessment and provides a valuable insight into what may be going on in your own body. But it is far from the most significant factor in whether you will develop heart disease. Isn't that good news?

I come from a family with a tremendously high risk of heart disease. My grandfather died of a massive heart attack the year before I was born. One of my uncles died of a heart attack in a Texas hospital emergency room while he was working as the ER physician that night. And he was in his mid-50s. I'm paying attention. But I'm not doing so by saying, "Well, I need to be a little more careful with my diet, I need to exercise a little more." You need to go far beyond that basic level of attention. You need to realistically understand your risk.

What about fasting blood sugar as an indicator of risk for heart disease? I think it's very important to know what your blood sugar levels are and to control them if need be. But in the Archimedes Study fully controlling fasting blood sugars for sixty years prevented only 9 percent of heart attacks.

It was the same with smoking. The study found that not smoking represented only a 9 percent reduction in the risk of having a heart attack. Many people think, *I don't smoke, so I'm not likely to develop heart disease.* No! Not smoking is important, just as family history and controlling blood sugars are important, but we need to understand the proportionality of risk. It's wise not to smoke, but don't think that not smoking, in and of itself, protects you enough. It doesn't.

There is a great deal of emphasis today on getting your LDL cholesterol level down. But in the Archimedes Study fully controlling LDL—the "bad" cholesterol—lowered the risk of heart attack by only 16 percent. What about HDL, the "good" cholesterol, the cholesterol that sucks the bad cholesterol out of the artery wall and takes it back to the liver to be detoxified and removed from the system? At this point, the study began finding some significant factors affecting risk of cardiovascular disease. Controlling HDL over the sixty years of the simulated aging process was found to prevent fully one-third of heart attacks. In addition, controlling the systolic blood pressure—the pressure in your circulatory system when the heart is contracting—so that it remained at youthful levels for the sixty years of the simulated study accounted for a 36 percent lower incidence of heart disease.

CORRECTING INSULIN RESISTANCE

But the single factor that beat all the others at reducing the risk of heart disease was correcting insulin resistance. In the Archimedes Study, controlling insulin resistance prevented 42 percent of all heart attacks! So let's look at the factors that are associated with insulin resistance—at the lab tests that best help us to understand if we have a problem in this area and, if so, to assess our risk, what we can do to reduce that risk, and even reverse it.

> Only if we know the truth of what is going on in our bodies can we address the reality and become motivated to take the necessary steps to deal with it.

Essentially, all type 2 diabetics, prediabetics, and many type 1 diabetics have insulin resistance. But it's my belief that the majority of individuals today with insulin resistance have neither diabetes nor prediabetes. They have resistance to insulin, so the pancreas makes a tremendous amount of insulin to offset their tendency to high blood sugars. That extra insulin controls their blood sugar problem.

That's why to test one's fasting blood sugar, as important as that test is, is a poor predictor of the underlying problem. A fasting blood sugar test is not sensitive enough; it doesn't catch the problem early enough. Checking blood sugars two hours after a sweet drink or a starchy meal is far more sensitive in indicating, not only diabetes and prediabetes, but the underlying insulin resistance.

One-half of those between the ages of 40 and 59 are at least prediabetic, as are two-thirds of those between the ages of 60 and 74. And among those older than 74, three-fourths are prediabetic.[6] Yet even these figures are only the tip of the iceberg. They don't account for the mammoth incidence of insulin resistance that is promoting many diseases, including hypertension, heart attacks, strokes,[7] Alzheimer's,[8] and cancers.[9]

High insulin often causes high blood pressure.[10] High insulin promotes low HDL, high triglycerides, and high LDL. High insulin tends to cause up-and-down changes in blood sugar which, in turn, often drive us to continue to smoke or participate in other unhealthy activities. For all these reasons, we need to be aware of any insulin resistance problems we may have and come to understand how to reverse it.

THE FIVE STAGES OF HIGH BLOOD SUGAR

	Stage 1	Stage 2	Stage 3	Stage 4	Stage 5
Time From Food Intake	Optimal Blood Sugar	High Blood Sugar	High Blood Sugar	Prediabetes	Advanced Prediabetes	Diabetes
Fasting	70-84	85-94	95-99	100-109	110-125	126+
1 hour	80-119	120-139	140-159	160-199	200+	
2 hours	80-99	100-119	120-139	140-159	160-199	200+

In 1996, while overseeing a government project to prevent, manage, and reverse diabetes on the island of Guam, I became concerned about the fact that people were developing complications of the disease even before they met the diagnostic criteria for diabetes. While discussing this with my colleagues, I recognized there was a great need for identifying categories of high blood sugars that precede actually having diabetes. And that is where the five stages of high blood sugar came from.

Stage 1. Blood sugars in Stage 1 represent the beginning of risk. A person with Stage 1 high blood sugars (fasting: 85-94) is probably already in a state of mild insulin resistance. If your fasting blood sugar is consistently in Stage 1, it would be wise to undergo a glucose tolerance test, which will give you a better understanding of your overall blood sugar control Because high blood sugars and insulin resistance increase the risk for cardiovascular disease, you should aggressively address these conditions and any other heart disease risk factors you may have. Stage 1 is the easiest to reverse. The earlier you take action, the better chance you have of being successful.

Stage 2. Blood sugars in this stage (fasting: 95-99) represent a heightened level of risk. Frequently, individuals with fasting blood sugars in the Stage 2 range who undergo a glucose tolerance test will be diagnosed with prediabetes or diabetes. If your fasting blood sugars are at Stage 2, it is very important to undergo additional testing and to aggressively address the underlying causes of your insulin resistance by following appropriate comprehensive lifestyle strategies.

Stage 3. This stage (fasting: 100-109) represents prediabetes. A fasting blood sugar of 100 is the threshold for prediabetes. If you have prediabetes, not only are you at high risk for developing diabetes in the future, but you are already at a much greater risk for developing heart disease. If you have prediabetes, it is crucial that you immediately take aggressive action to undergo additional testing and to address your blood sugars, insulin resistance, and heart disease risk factors.

Stage 4. If your blood sugars are at Stage 4 (fasting: 110-125) you are in advanced prediabetes and just a few points away from a diagnosis of full-blown diabetes. You are already at a dramatically increased risk for heart disease. At this stage it is urgent to do everything in your power to reverse your condition before it turns into full diabetes or a cardiovascular event. Be sure to undergo a glucose tolerance test, evaluate and address your other risk factors for heart disease, and begin implementing appropriate lifestyle strategies.

Stage 5. At Stage 5 (fasting: 126+) you meet the diagnostic criteria for diabetes. At this point, not only are you at an extremely increased risk for cardiovascular disease, but you are now also at risk for complications such as kidney failure, vision impairment or blindness, nerve damage, poor wound healing, amputations, and many other potential health problems.

Don't despair! Hope is available at every stage of high blood sugars.

Although blood sugar problems ideally should be identified as early as possible, even people who already have diabetes can take aggressive action to greatly improve, and even possibly reverse, the condition. Knowing these stages—and where you fit within them—gives you a critical educational approach to understanding your risk. Take advantage of knowing this information. If your blood sugars are high (stages 1 and 2), the pancreas is having to produce a lot of extra insulin. This is both good news and bad news. The good news, of course, is that the pancreas is working to control your blood sugar so that you don't have diabetes or prediabetes yet. But at what cost? That's the bad news—the extra insulin that the pancreas is having to produce puts you at risk for a multitude of health problems, including heart attacks and strokes.

WHO SHOULD GET TESTED: BETTER SAFE THAN SORRY

After more than twenty years of screening people for blood sugar imbalances, my clinical judgment leads me to believe that, when it comes to testing, *it's better to be safe than sorry.*

A mother recently came to my clinic with her two daughters—Emily, age fourteen, and Megan, age twelve. She wanted me to evaluate her health and the health of her girls. Emily was thin and lean. She didn't have any noticeable risk factors. Her mother was more interested in addressing Emily's acne problem. Because I like to look at the big picture when evaluating my patients, I also asked Emily about other aspects of her health. She mentioned that she sometimes felt fatigued. I did not suspect that she would have a problem with diabetes or prediabetes. She didn't have any risk factors, except that her grandmother was diabetic. Wondering if Emily might be hypoglycemic (have low blood sugar), I decided to order a four-hour glucose tolerance test (discussed later in this chapter).

When the results came back, I was surprised to discover that Emily was in the advanced stages of prediabetes. Her younger sister, Megan, was also prediabetic.

I applaud their mother for her willingness to have her family's health thoroughly evaluated. Their story is a reminder that diabetes and prediabetes can show up much earlier than age forty-five. People with a family history of diabetes—or with any of the other risk factors listed above—need to be intentional about early and regular screening. The earlier diabetes is caught, the better the chance of stopping it in its tracks.

It's important for patients and clinicians to realize that broad and thorough testing can identify conditions that would normally go unnoticed.

If you're willing to look at the big picture and test comprehensively, you're more likely to be able to detect and fix what's wrong. This chapter will provide you with practical information on how to evaluate your blood sugar levels to determine your risk for diabetes or prediabetes.

THE GLUCOSE TOLERANCE TEST

In my opinion, the glucose tolerance test is the *most* accurate and comprehensive test available for determining a predisposition for prediabetes or diabetes.[11] The glucose tolerance test shows how the body metabolizes and uses sugar (glucose) after it is ingested. It's not uncommon for people to have a fasting blood glucose level in the optimal range, but to be diagnosed as diabetic after an oral glucose tolerance test.

This test involves taking a fasting blood sugar level just before drinking a glucola drink—a concentrated, sweet drink that contains 75 grams of glucose. This is a metabolic stress test, designed to determine how your body responds to glucose.[12] Blood sugars are tested again at certain times after the drink is consumed. The results reveal the body's ability to control blood sugars effectively over time.

Two hours. The two-hour glucose tolerance test can be officially used to diagnose diabetes.[13] A clinician will test the fasting blood sugar before a glucola drink is given, give the glucola drink, and then test the blood sugar again two hours after the drink is finished. A blood sugar level of 200 or higher after two hours is a definitive diagnosis of diabetes. A blood sugar level of 140 to 199 is prediabetes.[14]

The story of Emily, the fourteen-year-old patient mentioned previously, illustrates the value of the two-hour glucose test. Although I didn't suspect that Emily had a problem with prediabetes or diabetes, I ordered a glucose tolerance test to check for hypoglycemia. Emily's fasting blood glucose was 73—a perfect level. However, I was surprised to discover that her two-hour glucose tolerance level was 195—just five points away from an official diagnosis of diabetes. Emily had advanced prediabetes. This condition would have gone undetected for years, possibly even decades, if I had considered only her fasting glucose level. The two-hour test revealed that Emily had a problem and gave her the opportunity to begin addressing her condition at an early age, before the condition had time to progress.

Because an official diagnosis for prediabetes or diabetes can be determined by either the fasting blood glucose test or the two-hour glucose tolerance test, these are the two most common tests that clinicians use.[15] But when I perform a two-hour glucose tolerance test, I also like to check the blood sugar at one hour.

One hour. Although the one-hour glucose tolerance test is not part of the official criteria used to diagnose diabetes, it also provides valuable information. This test is more sensitive in detecting early tendencies toward blood sugar problems than are the fasting and two-hour tests. For this reason, I recommend that any time a glucose tolerance test is done, it should include a one-hour reading.

> Researchers have determined that a blood sugar level of 155 or higher one hour after consuming 75 grams of glucose is an independent risk factor for cardiovascular disease.[16] Since the primary focus of diagnosing diabetes and prediabetes is to help prevent and lower the risk of cardiovascular disease, it is important to pay attention to this test.

Emily's younger sister, Megan, is a good example of someone who benefited from the one-hour glucose tolerance test. Because Emily's and Megan's mom wanted me to thoroughly evaluate both of her daughters, I ordered a glucose tolerance test for Megan as well. Megan's fasting blood sugar was 79—an optimal level. Her two-hour level was 100—also a normal level. If that were all the information we had, it would have appeared that Megan had optimal blood sugars. However, I also ordered a one-hour level to be drawn. When the results came back, I realized that Megan did in fact have a blood sugar problem. Her one-hour level was 200.

Because the one-hour test is not diagnostic, Megan could not be officially diagnosed as "prediabetic." However, this test showed me that she was experiencing blood sugar spikes after meals, which, if left untreated, would cause serious damage to her body over time. Thankfully, the one-hour test caught the problem, and Megan learned how to manage her blood sugars after meals. Megan was very fortunate to have learned about her risk at such a young age. This gave her the opportunity to take control and to avoid serious complications in the future.

THE FOUR-HOUR GLUCOSE TOLERANCE TEST

Although the two-hour glucose tolerance test is the most sensitive test for detecting prediabetes, diabetes, and insulin resistance, it is also beneficial to check the blood sugar levels at three and four hours. This provides valuable insights into adrenal function and any tendency to low blood sugars—clinically referred to as reactive hypoglycemia. I almost always recommend the four-hour glucose tolerance test that checks blood sugars at fasting, one-half hour, and at one, two, three, and four hours after drinking the 75 grams of sugary drink. This gives a four-hour "glycemic curve," showing how high, and then how low, the blood sugars spike and dip between 8:00 A.M. and 12:00 noon on the morning of testing. To further understand the underlying metabolic function I strongly recommend also testing the insulin levels during the GTT at fasting and at one and two hours.

PEPSI®-JELLY BEAN CHALLENGE

There is a do-it-yourself way to perform a modified glucose tolerance test at home. I call this the "Pepsi®-Jelly Bean Challenge."

Several years ago, I was reading an article in a medical journal that described an alternate method of doing the glucose tolerance test.[17] Typically, all pregnant women are given a glucose tolerance test at twenty-eight weeks to screen for gestational diabetes. Many pregnant women dislike the sugary sweet drink and have trouble getting or keeping it down. To make it easier on them, some clinics began allowing them to eat jelly beans instead of drinking the glucola drink.

This idea appealed to me for several reasons. I realized that people would be more eager to do the test if they were able to eat jelly beans or other sugary snacks. This would also give them the flexibility of testing at home, using their own glucose meter and food or drinks. In addition, it would wake them up to the fact that their favorite snacks and drinks could seriously affect their blood sugars.

I have had many patients take the glucose tolerance test with the glucola drink and test positive for diabetes or prediabetes. These patients tend to minimize their risk, saying, "Well, of *course* my blood sugar went up after drinking that drink. But I would never drink something *that* sweet on a regular basis!" For this reason, I developed the Pepsi®-Jelly Bean Challenge.

I named it after Pepsi's popular marketing campaign, the "Pepsi® Challenge." But the goal of the Pepsi®-Jelly Bean Challenge isn't to determine whether Pepsi® or Coke® tastes better. It's to show people how either of these drinks— along with any other sugary drinks or snacks—affect their blood sugars.

To take the Pepsi®-Jelly Bean Challenge, get your favorite soda or sugary drink and your favorite starchy snacks (cookies, candy, crackers, etc.). After checking and recording your fasting blood glucose level, eat your snacks and drink your drink. One hour later, and two hours later, check and record your blood glucose levels again. Then use the information recorded above in the section, **THE FIVE STAGES OF HIGH BLOOD SUGAR** (pg. 251) to determine whether you have prediabetes or diabetes. The success of the Pepsi®-Jelly Bean Challenge is illustrated by the story of Chris.

Several years ago, I was teaching a university wellness class. Knowing that more than 20 percent of these students probably had prediabetes or diabetes,[18] I wanted to make them aware of the importance of blood sugar management.

I asked everyone to bring their favorite sugary and starchy snacks to our next class period—sodas, juice, cookies, candy, crackers, etc. Each person was to bring 75 to 100 grams of sugar or starch, which is 300 to 400 calories.

When the next class period came, the students were prepared. At the beginning of class, the students ate and drank their sugary snacks. About an hour later, I had the staff from my clinic test the students' blood sugar levels. Quite a few students were surprised to discover that their blood sugars were running high. However, one young man was deeply concerned.

Chris approached me at the end of class looking utterly defeated. "I don't know what I'm going to do," he said. "My blood sugar is 350. I didn't even know that I had a problem." Working his way through college, twenty-five-year-old Chris was under a lot of stress. He was about fifty pounds overweight and smoked two packs of cigarettes a day.

"Let's check it again once it's been two hours since your snack," I told him. We did, and it was well above 200.

Although Chris had a family history of diabetes, he was young and didn't think that it could happen to him. Thankfully, he had enrolled in this required wellness class and discovered that he had a problem. Chris became highly motivated to address his condition. He remembered his Uncle Joe, who had had his leg amputated from out-of-control diabetes, and his grandfather who had gone blind before passing away. He wanted to overcome his genetic risk and outsmart the disease.

Throughout the rest of the class, I worked with Chris to address his diabetes. He started exercising every day. He started eating well. His energy returned. By the end of ten weeks, Chris had lost thirty pounds, stopped smoking, and dramatically improved his blood sugar levels. In fact, he no longer fit the criteria for diabetes. Because of a simple Pepsi®-Jelly Bean Challenge and Chris' motivation to change—his health had been transformed.

DIRECTIONS FOR THE PEPSI®-JELLY BEAN CHALLENGE
NECESSARY SUPPLIES:

Blood glucose monitoring kit and supplies

Sugary, starchy snacks equaling 75 to 100 grams of starch or sugar total (i.e. 300 to 400 calories from sugar).

These snacks can include:
Sodas (not diet), juice, jelly beans, candy, crackers, or sugar cookies
*Note: Avoid eating any significant amount of fat or protein.

PERFORMING THE TEST:

1. Take and record your fasting blood glucose level. (Although technically a fasting glucose level is obtained after twelve hours of not eating or drinking anything except water, for the sake of this test you need to wait only three or more hours. By this time, blood sugar levels will be very close to fasting levels.

2. Eat and drink your sugary snacks and beverages.

3. After one hour, take and record your blood glucose level.

4. After two hours, take and record your blood glucose level.

5. Evaluate your fasting, one-hour, and two-hour blood glucose levels according to the information given above in the section, **THE FIVE STAGES OF HIGH BLOOD SUGAR** to determine whether your blood sugars are compromised.

Note: If you don't want to drink soda or candy, you can eat a starchy meal such as spaghetti or pancakes. Just be sure that the majority of the calories are coming from carbohydrates, not protein or fat. (For example, if you're eating spaghetti, avoid eating Alfredo sauce or meatballs. Stick with just the spaghetti. If you're eating pancakes, avoid adding butter or eggs or any other protein at the same time.)

Sometimes when I suggest the Pepsi®-Jelly Bean Challenge to patients, they don't think it will apply to them. They assume that because they don't regularly eat sugary snacks or drink soda, they don't have a blood sugar problem. It's important to note that many starchy foods eaten on a regular basis can cause blood sugar spikes. I tell these patients that they can pick their favorite 100 percent juice and whole wheat crackers. The test results will still reveal any tendency toward high blood sugar.

The Pepsi®-Jelly Bean Challenge evaluates more than just the effect of junk food on blood sugars; it provides information on how the body processes glucose in general.

TESTING INSULIN

The pancreas is a six-inch-long gland that lies slightly behind the stomach, level with the small intestine. It is shaped like a tall, thin pear, lying on its side. The pancreas gland has multiple functions. It secretes digestive enzymes into the small intestine to help break down food. It is also responsible for the secretion of several different hormones, including insulin. Insulin is produced inside the beta cells in the pancreas.

People with type 1 diabetes have sustained damage to the beta cells of the pancreas and are no longer able to produce a significant amount of insulin. People with type 2 diabetes typically still have a functional pancreas, but their muscles and tissues have become resistant to the insulin their pancreas produces. One way to measure pancreatic function is to have your insulin levels tested.

You already know it's important to test the amount of *sugar* in your blood, but it can also be important to test the amount of *insulin* in your blood.[19] If you are not taking insulin injections, your natural insulin level can reveal how hard your pancreas is working to stabilize your blood sugars.

If blood sugars are high but insulin levels are extremely low, especially after a meal, this indicates the presence of type 1 diabetes. The pancreas has been damaged. If insulin levels are high, this indicates that the pancreas is producing plenty of insulin, but that the body is resistant to that insulin. Often, people with type 2 diabetes have hyperinsulinemia,[20] which means that the pancreas is working extra hard to produce more insulin than is usually required, in an attempt to force glucose into cells. Eventually, the pancreas will become fatigued. When blood sugars are running high, even a normal insulin level may suggest that the pancreas is losing its ability to produce insulin.

High insulin levels increase the risk of multiple diseases including hypertension,[21] heart disease,[22] obesity,[23] prostate cancer,[24] colon cancer,[25] breast cancer,[26] infertility,[27] and Alzheimer's Disease.[28]

Because all of these conditions can be associated with high insulin levels, having your insulin tested not only provides information about your pancreatic function and your diabetes, but may also help you determine your risk for these other diseases.

THE FASTING INSULIN TEST

The fasting insulin test can be taken at the same time as the fasting blood glucose test. It measures the amount of insulin in the blood after not eating since the night before. This test is not performed for people who are taking insulin injections because the injected insulin would combine with the insulin the body produces naturally, which would skew the results.

A result of 5 μIU/mL for this test is excellent—many young athletes fit in this category. A healthy target range is 7 μIU/mL or lower, while a result of 10 μIU/mL or higher indicates increased risk

I was first introduced to the importance of insulin testing more than twenty years ago when I listened to a lecture by Nancy Bohannon, M.D. Dr. Bohannon directs the Cardiovascular Risk Reduction Program at St. Luke's Hospital in San Francisco. In this lecture, she shared the importance of testing insulin levels to determine risk for heart disease. She suggested that insulin levels should be under 10 μIU/mL.[29]

Dr. Bohannon's lecture motivated me to begin testing insulin levels in my patients. If a patient's fasting insulin level was above 10, I determined that it indicated increased risk. If the level was below 10, I assumed that no risk was present. However, after carefully observing my patients and reviewing the research on this topic, I concluded that any level above seven suggested increased risk. Some functional medicine experts are even suggesting that levels should be under 5 μIU/mL.[30]

> If your fasting insulin level is high, you can take action to address your insulin resistance and reduce your risk for disease. The lifestyle strategies in this book are designed to increase your body's sensitivity to insulin and to stabilize both insulin levels and blood sugar levels.

TWO-HOUR INSULIN LEVEL TEST

Whenever I order a glucose tolerance test, I recommend a two-hour insulin level test at the same time as the two-hour blood sugar level. Sometimes people who are fasting show healthy insulin levels, but when sugar is in the system those levels rise dramatically.

MEASURING PANCREATIC FUNCTION: THE C-PEPTIDE TEST

If you're already taking insulin because you have diabetes and your body cannot produce enough insulin on its own to control your blood sugar, a C-peptide test can be beneficial. This test tells whether the pancreas is still healthy, and it can help determine if there is a possibility that you could minimize your insulin medications over the next one to three months. If your pancreas is still healthy, getting on the right program and following the right wellness strategies can dramatically help you reverse your diabetes.

If the test shows that the C-peptide level is very low, you will probably need to continue insulin medication, at least for some time. The objective, in this case, is not getting off insulin medication; the objective is how to optimize your healing potential, minimize your risk of heart attack, kidney failure, amputation, or blindness.

> When a person develops diabetes, it is important to determine whether they have type 1 or type 2. As we have seen, one way to test this is by evaluating insulin levels. Pancreatic function can also be determined by the C-peptide test.[31]

People with diabetes sometimes do not know whether they have type 1 or type 2. Patients may be prescribed insulin without knowing whether they are naturally producing any insulin or not. But once they are taking insulin injections, an insulin test won't reliably determine whether or not their pancreas is producing insulin. The test cannot tell the difference between insulin that's being produced by the pancreas and insulin that's being injected.

The C-peptide test solves this problem by evaluating natural insulin production another way. C-peptide is a protein produced by the pancreas. The pancreas releases this protein at the same time it releases insulin. For every molecule of insulin released, a molecule of C-peptide is also released. Because the level of C-peptide corresponds with the level of insulin, this test can be used to evaluate how much insulin the pancreas is producing.

NORMAL USE OF THE C-PEPTIDE TEST

The C-peptide test is normally used to help determine whether patients who are taking insulin injections have type 1 or type 2 diabetes.[32] [33] If the C-peptide level is normal or high, this means that the pancreas is producing a normal or high amount of insulin, indicating that type 2 diabetes is present, which is most frequently characterized by insulin resistance.

If the C-peptide test is very low, this means that the pancreas is producing very little—if any—insulin. This indicates type 1 diabetes, which is caused by inadequate insulin production.

EXPERIMENTAL/INNOVATIVE USE OF THE C-PEPTIDE TEST

The C-peptide test can reveal more information than just which type of diabetes is present. Because this test measures how well the pancreas is producing insulin, it actually tells how much damage has occurred to the pancreatic tissue and what the long-term chances are that a person will be able to fully control their blood sugars without the use of insulin or other medications.

Recently, a group of lifestyle medicine physicians developed a new, experimental test to evaluate the probability that diabetic patients taking multiple medications would eventually be able to control their blood sugars without medications after several months of intensive lifestyle therapy.[34] This test is an adaptation of the stimulated C-peptide test.

To perform the test, patients were given a sugary drink or carbohydrate-rich meal (similar to a glucose tolerance test). Approximately an hour later, after blood sugars had increased from the meal and the pancreas was the most likely to be producing insulin and C-peptide, the C-peptide level was measured. The amount of C-peptide in the blood revealed how effective the pancreas was at secreting insulin and C-peptide in response to rising blood sugars.

The team of physicians developed criteria to explain what the results of the stimulated C-peptide levels mean.

Interpreting the stimulated C-peptide test. A result of less than 2 ng/ mL indicates that the pancreas is severely damaged and that there is only an estimated 5 percent chance of controlling blood sugars through lifestyle interventions alone. A reading of 2-4 ng/mL means that the pancreas has undergone some damage, but is still functioning. There is a fifty/fifty chance of controlling blood sugars without insulin or other medications. A result of 4 ng/mL or higher means that the pancreas is functioning well. There is an estimated 95 percent chance that blood sugars can eventually be controlled through lifestyle interventions alone, without insulin or other medication.

It's important to note that this was simply an experimental model and these are not official criteria. However, I believe that this new approach is a valuable way to determine the extent of pancreatic damage and to predict whether patients will be able to control their blood sugars with lifestyle approaches alone—or whether they may need to supplement their lifestyle changes with insulin.

> The lines between type 1 diabetes and type 2 diabetes are not always as clear as we once thought. Many people who initially develop type 2 diabetes sustain damage to the pancreas after years of high blood sugars and unhealthy choices. Over time, the ability of the pancreas to produce insulin becomes more and more compromised.

By using these experimental guidelines to evaluate pancreatic function, we better understand a person's long-term prognosis. This helps us develop a realistic treatment plan.

TESTING FOR FERRITIN

Iron and ferritin, a storage form of iron, should be measured in everybody. It's not usually part of a standard physical or included in the usual blood testing protocol, but it's a test that everyone should have. Why? Because so many people are either low or high in iron. If you're too low, you are at risk for depression and fatigue. But a high iron or ferritin level can promote diabetes,[35] heart attacks, formation of plaque in the arteries, and cancers.[36]

Several years ago, Todd came to see me. He was a school teacher who had been diagnosed with diabetes more than fifteen years earlier. Todd explained to me that he was taking his medications regularly and had come in only because his wife kept insisting that he see me. Being very fond of steak and meat in general, he wasn't eager for me to evaluate his diet.

Understanding his concern, I suggested that we first review his old lab tests and see if he was missing any that could suggest how he might further improve his health. Even though his blood sugars had been fairly well controlled, Todd had suffered a retinal detachment in one eye, leaving him partially blind. It seemed to me that something besides high blood sugars was contributing to his health complications.

Todd agreed to take the additional lab tests outlined in this chapter. A week later he came back for a full review of his new lab tests. To his surprise, Todd's stored form of iron, called ferritin, was thirteen times higher that it ideally should have been. Instead of an optimal level of 70 to 110, Todd's ferritin was nearly 1,400! Even though he had been diabetic for many years, he had never been encouraged to have his iron and ferritin checked. I called Todd's family doctor to discuss the new finding, and we both agreed that Todd would benefit from seeing a Hematologist who specialized in blood disorders. Todd had a fairly common genetic disorder that caused an abnormal buildup of iron in his blood.

This buildup of iron had likely been a key trigger to his diabetes and eye-nerve damage. By getting the broader testing done, Todd was now able to follow the simple medical and nutritional strategies for normalizing ferritin. I believe Todd would have suffered a stroke or heart attack within a few years if he had not been properly diagnosed. In addition, Todd is now much less likely to develop cancer.

It's easy to regulate the amount of iron in the body so that it is neither too high nor too low—if you know about it. That is why testing is so important. Over and over, I've seen individuals who were willing to do broad testing, uncover problems that would have led to an early death if they hadn't learned about them in time.

THE REST OF ANN'S STORY

Let's come back to Ann's story. You'll remember that she was afraid she had breast cancer, but it turned out to be a benign lipoma, a fatty growth. However, the broad range of testing that we did gave Ann an opportunity to step back and evaluate her health in a comprehensive way.

Of course, she had been ecstatic when the CT scan dismissed her fears of breast cancer. Her first reaction had been to say, "That's great! There is nothing to worry about, and I can go on with my life." She had been focused on that one big concern, and now she didn't have to worry about that. But she had done all these comprehensive laboratory tests, so she decided she might as well sit down and see what they said about her health.

As I looked at her test results, I was impressed by how many "potholes" she had—unnoticed, hidden factors that negatively affected her health in significant ways. I get excited when I see potholes. Why? Because they are opportunities. They've been there all along; you just haven't been aware of them.

> Of course, you can just keep falling into potholes, keep getting injured, and keep crawling back out of them if you can. Or you can fill them up. We can remove them as an obstacle to your health. I get excited about helping people see what's really going on in their bodies, the hidden causes of disease.

As I looked at Ann's chart, everything was out of whack. Her thyroid was out of control. Her thyroid antibodies which should have been under 60, were nearly 1,000! The actual thyroid hormone was low; the reverse T3, the inactivated form of thyroid hormone was very high. She had no clue there was anything wrong with her thyroid. The only reason she had all this lab work done was because of the lump in her armpit. She had taken my advice to test broadly, and the result was that she was finding out things about her body and her health that she had never known.

I told her, "Ann, you need to discuss these results with your primary care doctor. I'll help with the big picture." I believe it's important for everyone to have a healthcare team that they can rely on to give them good information and feedback. But the head of that healthcare team, the person in charge, is *you!* You are personally in charge of your own board of health. And if you choose not to accept that responsibility, you aren't going to enjoy optimal health. You're putting yourself at critical risk.

Ann had been like so many people who say, "I'm not going to get lab work done unless it's absolutely necessary. I'm going to avoid any unnecessary procedures." But by doing so, they deny themselves critical information that they need to know in order to establish powerful strategies to reverse unhealthful conditions. Fortunately, Ann was willing to look at the big picture and follow through on the results of the testing we did. She was able to step back and evaluate her health comprehensively, so that she could develop sound strategies for her personal health and wellness.

Work with your healthcare team to determine the tests that best fit your goals and needs. Not everyone needs the same tests. Below are some additional tests you should consider as you take charge of your health.

THE COMPREHENSIVE METABOLIC PROFILE (CMP)

The comprehensive metabolic profile, the CMP, gives us a lot of information. It's a standard test on most physical exams. It gives a broad review of the body's systems, including fasting blood glucose, blood electrolyte/mineral levels, kidney, liver, and digestive function, protein status, immune parameters, and basic detox function. A detailed description follows on the next four pages.

THE COMPLETE BLOOD COUNT (CBC)

The Complete Blood Count is the main blood panel that reviews the status of the red blood cells (RBC), white blood cells (WBC), and their respective components. The CBC provides clues to many aspect of health including tendency to anemia, acute infection, and immune status.

B12 AND FOLATE

If you're already taking Vitamin B12 and folate, it's probably not going to be too helpful to test for these items. But if you haven't been taking any supplements, it's beneficial to determine the levels of these things in your body. We know from many studies that if you're in the low normal range for Vitamin B12, you have a dramatically increased risk of Alzheimer's disease.[37] That alone should be reason enough to pay attention to Vitamin B12. But Vitamin B12 has other far-reaching influences on your health as well.

Comprehensive Metabolic Profile (CMP)	Reference Ranges*
Glucose (fasting or non-fasting) Sugar in the blood **Low numbers indicate:** Hypoglycemia, liver disease, adrenal insufficiency, excess insulin **High numbers indicate:** Hyperglycemia, certain types of diabetes, prediabetes, pancreatitis, hyperthyroidism	70-99 mg/dL (fasting) 70-125 mg/dL (non-fasting)
Sodium (Na) An electrolyte which keeps your body in balance **Low numbers indicate:** Use of diuretics, diarrhea, adrenal insufficiency **High numbers indicate:** Kidney dysfunction, dehydration, Cushing's syndrome	136-144 mEq/L
Potassium (K) An electrolyte and mineral **Low numbers indicate:** Use of diuretics or corticosteroids (such as prednisone or cortisone) **High numbers indicate:** Acute or chronic kidney failure, Addison's disease, diabetes, dehydration	3.7-5.2 mEq/L
Chloride (Cl) An electrolyte **Low numbers indicate:** Emphysema, chronic lung disease **High numbers indicate:** Dehydration, Cushing's syndrome, kidney disease	96-106 mmol/L

Comprehensive Metabolic Profile (CMP)	Reference Ranges*
Carbon dioxide (bicarbonate) (CO2) Gaseous waste product from metabolism **Low numbers indicate:** Kidney disease, certain toxic exposures, severe infection **High numbers indicate:** Lung diseases, including COPD	20-29 mmol/L
BUN (blood urea nitrogen) A chemical waste produced by muscle metabolism **Low numbers indicate:** Malnutrition **High numbers indicate:** Liver or kidney disease, heart failure	7-20 mg/dL
Creatinine An electrolyte which keeps your body in balance **Low numbers indicate:** Low muscle mass, malnutrition **High numbers indicate:** Chronic or temporary decrease in kidney function	0.8-1.4 mg/dL
BUN/creatinine ratio **Low numbers indicate:** Malnutrition **High numbers indicate:** Blood in bowels, kidney obstruction, dehydration	10:1 to 20:1
Calcium (Ca) A mineral stored in the hard part of bones **Low numbers indicate:** Calcium, magnesium, or Vitamin D deficiency; malnutrition; pancreatitis; neurological disorders **High numbers indicate:** Kidney disease, hyperparathyroidism, cancer, excess vitamin D intake	8.5-10.9 mg/dL
Magnesium (Mg) An electrolyte **Low numbers indicate:** Diabetes, high blood calcium levels, kidney disease, pancreatitis, hypoparathyroidism **High numbers indicate:** Dehydration, Addison's disease, hyperparathyroidism, hypothyroidism, kidney failure	1.8-2.6 mEq/L

Comprehensive Metabolic Profile (CMP)	Reference Ranges*
Protein (total) Chains of amino acids essential for the growth and repair of cells **Low numbers indicate:** Malnutrition, liver disease, kidney disease **High numbers indicate:** Liver disease, kidney disease, dehydration, multiple myeloma, WM	6.3-7.9 g/dL
Albumin Protein that keeps fluid from leaking out of blood vessels and that nourishes tissues and transports nutrients through the body **Low numbers indicate:** Malnutrition, liver disease, kidney disease **High numbers indicate:** Dehydration	3.9-5.0 g/dL
Globulin Alpha, beta, and gamma proteins; some are produced by the liver and others by the immune system **Low numbers indicate:** Malnutrition, liver disease, kidney disease **High numbers indicate:** Multiple myeloma, WM, leukemia, rheumatoid arthritis, lupus, and other autoimmune diseases	2.0-3.5 g/dL
Albumin/globulin ratio **Low numbers indicate:** Multiple myeloma, WM, autoimmune diseases, liver disease, kidney disease **High numbers indicate:** Certain genetic conditions, some leukemias, liver dysfunction, hypogammaglobulinemia	1.7-2.2
Bilirubin (direct or total) A pigment in the bile, a digestive fluid produced by the liver **Low numbers indicate:** Generally not a concern **High numbers indicate:** Liver disease, bile duct disorder, red cell destruction	0-0.3 mg/dL (direct) 0.3-1.9 mg/dL (total)

Comprehensive Metabolic Profile (CMP)	Reference Ranges*
Alkaline phosphatase (ALP) Enzyme found in the liver and bones **Low numbers indicate:** Malnutrition **High numbers indicate:** Paget's disease or certain cancers that spread to bone, bile duct obstruction, liver cancer	44-147 IU/L
Alanine amino-transferase (ALT) Enzyme found mostly in the liver **Low numbers indicate:** Generally not a concern **High numbers indicate:** Certain toxins such as excess acetaminophen or alcohol, hepatitis	8-37 IU/L
Aspartate amino-transferase (AST) Enzyme found in liver, muscle, and other tissues **Low numbers indicate:** Generally not a concern **High numbers indicate:** Excess acetaminophen, hepatitis muscle injury	10-34 IU/L
Glomerular filtration rate (GFR) Checks how well the kidneys are working by estimating how much blood passes through the glomeruli (filters) of the kidneys each minute **Low numbers indicate:** Chronic kidney disease or kidney failure; GFR decreases progressively with age **High numbers indicate:** Generally not a concern	90-120 mL/min/1.73 m2

Reference ranges can vary by age, sex, methods of testing, and other factors. There are no nationally established reference ranges for CMP and CBC values; instead, each laboratory tests a population and establishes its own reference ranges. Therefore, the reference ranges quoted are only approximate. The reference ranges presented here are U.S. measurements. Other country values can often be located online.

HOMOCYSTEINE[38]

Homocysteine is an amino acid that is converted from the amino acid, methionine, which comes from our food and which can then be converted into the amino acid cysteine. Cysteine is critical for glutathione production and the day-to-day detoxification process that occurs in the liver. When the converting enzymes have inadequate access to activating vitamins, homocysteine will accumulate to unhealthy levels. Higher than optimal levels of homocysteine are associated with increased risk of heart disease, Alzheimer's,[39] dementia, depression, osteoporosis, kidney disease, certain cancers, and many other health concerns.

A blood test for homocysteine is valuable as it helps us understand our functional requirement for key nutrients that strongly influence our body's natural ability to detoxify, thus keeping the immune system in balance.

When homocysteine builds up in the blood, it becomes toxic to many body systems.[40] Optimal levels are less than 7.2. Levels above 9.0 are strongly suggestive of a functional Vitamin B12 deficiency and possibly of an inadequate intake of Folate and Vitamin B6.

VITAMIN D[41]

Vitamin D testing is a critical part of your health tune up and one that is very easy to "fix." Low levels of Vitamin D dramatically increase the risk of catching a cold or flu through the winter months.[42] New studies show that low Vitamin D levels are associated with more than double the risk of developing Alzheimer's.[43] Studies estimate that 35 percent of all cancers could be eliminated if we optimized our blood level of Vitamin D.[44] Low levels greatly increase the risk of infections, pneumonia, autoimmune disease, diabetes, and neurological and mental health problems. Don't think that being in the sun regularly eliminates your need to test Vitamin D levels. Even though I am a beach and sun lover, my Vitamin D level has been as low as 25. Get tested and then take enough Vitamin D to achieve a 50 to 100 ng/dL on your blood test.

FULL MALE OR FEMALE HORMONE PROFILE

Young and old alike often benefit from a thorough review of hormones. Natural and nutritional protocols can dramatically improve the balance and function of hormones, but the first step is learning whether certain hormones are too high or too low, especially in relation to each other. For example, a woman's estradiol many not be elevated, but when combined with a very low progesterone level, there is a problem of estrogen dominance.

> Hormones can be effectively measured using blood, urine, or saliva. I typically recommend a combination of blood and saliva. Depending on age and health goals, the hormones most often useful for testing include cortisol, DHEA sulfate, total and free testosterone, estradiol, total estrogens, progesterone, and pregnenolone.

When using blood to test hormones it is also helpful to test the levels of albumin and of sex hormone binding globulin (SHBG). High levels of these two proteins can bind and inactivate sex hormones even though the hormones themselves test at normal levels in the blood.

THE STICKY BLOOD SUGAR TEST—THE HEMOGLOBIN A1C TEST

The hemoglobin A1C test is an important means of determining whether you are prediabetic or diabetic. But it also gives significant insights into whether you are insulin resistant. This test looks at how much your blood sugar spikes after each meal. If your blood sugars are spiking after a meal, that means your body is having to produce more insulin to try to control that excess blood sugar. And this high insulin is a major factor in heart attacks and strokes.

In Chapter 9 I referred to the hemoglobin A1C test as the "sticky blood sugar test." Is your blood sugar spiking after meals? How often does that happen? How high does it go? That's what the sticky blood sugar test tells us. You want the results of this test to be at least under 5.7 percent which is the beginning of prediabetes. Type 2 diabetes or even Type 1 diabetes can be defined as a level of 6.5 percent or higher. The more sugar that sticks to cells when the blood sugar spikes after meals, the more damage is done. That's why I refer to this test as a pathology test. It's not just a measure of how high your blood sugars have been over the past few months. It's actually a direct measurement of how much pathological damage has been done to the tissues of your body by high blood sugars.

When sugar sticks to the cells, this is actually an irreversible glycosylation, or glazing, of sugar to the protein molecules in the tissues. This drastically damages the functionality of the cells and therefore activates the immune system against those tissues.

This is why high blood sugars cause damage to all systems of the body and represent a serious risk factor for complications in your circulation, kidneys, eyesight, and your nervous system. Fortunately, over time we can actually reverse the irreversible. As we begin to control blood sugars both before and after meals, the old sugar-glazed cells die and are removed by immune cells. The new cells are no longer being exposed to this damage from high blood sugars, so a decrease in the hemoglobin A1C is noticeable within a few weeks. This is what allows for dramatic drops in the A1C level with two to three months.

Optimal levels of hemoglobin A1C are 5.0 percent or a little less. I find that the vast majority of people are not at optimal levels. Most "apparently healthy" people are somewhere between optimal (5.0 percent) and prediabetes (5.7 percent). Every percentage point that the hemoglobin A1C lab test goes above 5.0 percent represents a 37 percent increased risk of nerve damage, a 37 percent increased risk of vision loss and kidney disease, and a 21 percent increased risk of premature death.[45]

I see patients whose hemoglobin A1C test is 10 percent, 11 percent, or higher. Can you imagine how excited and thrilled they are when only two or three months later their test result is at 6.0 percent or better? How were they able to do that? They did it by first embracing the diagnosis and recognizing their problem. Instead of saying, "It's too far gone now; I probably have irreversible damage," they recognized that the body will heal itself if given half a chance. It's exciting to see what a consistent, sound wellness program can do.

GOING BEYOND THE STANDARD LIPID PROFILE

The standard lipid profile looks at the total cholesterol, the LDL cholesterol, the HDL, and triglycerides. This is an important test, and we know that these cholesterol levels are linked closely to cardiovascular health. But altogether they represent only about 50 percent of the risk of having a heart attack.[46] That's why it is important to go beyond the standard lipid profile and look at advanced cardiovascular risk factors. One way to do this is the Lp-PLA2 test, commonly called the PLAC test, that measures the enzymes being released by plaque cells in your artery walls. That's a valuable test. The goal is to keep the Lp-PLA2 level well under 200ng/dL.[47] I frequently find that patients with completely normal cholesterol levels have elevated plaque levels. Everything else seems to be okay, but their PLAC levels are high. That means the artery wall itself is inflamed and plaque ridden. If you had that condition, wouldn't you want to know?

Things we don't know *can* hurt us. Risk factors that we continue to avoid learning about *will* hurt us. And the exciting thing is that these risk factors are often completely reversible!

THE CARDIAC CRP TEST

The high sensitivity CRP (hs-CRP), or the "cardiac CRP" as it's also called, is another general test for inflammation and is part of the Hunter Heart Profile (see Chapter 3). If you score high on the cardiac CRP test (above 2.0 mg/L) and you're also high (above 200 ng/dL) on the PLAC test, you are facing an eleven-fold greater risk for stroke![48]

Most people don't realize that the standard lipid profile and the metabolic profile actually have very little predictive value for TIAs and strokes. They have predictive value for heart disease, but not for strokes. The PLAC test has a predictive value for stroke directly.[49] So do the other tests that measure inflammation.

You should be taking advantage of these tests as you move forward in planning a comprehensive wellness program that will allow you to reverse these risk factors.

The normal range for the cardiac CRP is 1 to 3 mg/L. But you don't want to be just "normal" when it comes to risk for cardiovascular disease! According to studies done at Harvard University, once your cardiac CRP level is above 1, you're already above the 40th percentile.[50] That's not good. You don't ever want to be at average risk for cardiovascular risk factors. Why? Because in today's world it's "average"—it's "expected"—to have heart disease. That's why it's so important to have the cardiac CRP test early and begin to reverse as many of the risk factors as possible. You want to keep the level of inflammation as close to zero as you possibly can. Normal or average risk for heart disease is actually unacceptably high risk!

THE ADVANCED CARDIAC PROFILE

There are three other tests that are included in the advanced cardiac profile. The first is the sticky LDL cholesterol test. This test measures the level of lipoprotein (a), also known as "sticky LDL cholesterol." It's so sticky that it dramatically increases the tendency for plaque formation. In part, a high level of lipoprotein (a) is a genetic risk factor.[51] That means an individual with this problem is probably going to have to work on it throughout his or her life. If you have elevated levels of sticky cholesterol—30 mg/dL or higher—that represents an increased risk of heart disease. The amount of plaque-forming cholesterol contained in sticky cholesterol is ten times more predictive of premature heart disease than is regular LDL cholesterol.[52] So it's important to know your sticky cholesterol level. There are some specific nutritional strategies that work to lower this risk factor.

Another test in the advanced cardiac profile is the test for small, dense LDL (sd-LDL). LDL is the "bad" cholesterol, but a variant of LDL—sd-LDL—is even worse. Cholesterol comes in different sizes. There are large, fluffy LDL particles, and then there are smaller and smaller ones. The small dense LDL (sd-LDL) particles are so tiny they can cross right into the artery wall, causing irritation and promoting plaque buildup. If it is determined that your levels of sd-LDL are elevated, you can't just take statin medications as a way of combating it. In fact, many of the statin medications actually *increase* some forms of sticky cholesterol and sd-LDL cholesterol.[53]

A third test in the advanced cardiac profile deals with HDL cholesterol.

This is the "good" cholesterol. The standard lipid profile includes the HDL "healthy" cholesterol, but there is a more specific form of HDL called HDL2b—the most protective type of HDL.[54] In general, an HDL2b of more than 25 percent is considered protective for cardiovascular risk. Of course, it's important to look at the combined influence of all the cardiovascular risk factors.

Having a higher HDL2b is a good thing. However, if one or more of the other risk factors are present, we need to establish specific nutritional and lifestyle strategies to resolve each one independently and then retest in six to eight weeks to see if our current plan is working or if it needs to be adjusted.

> Each one of these advanced tests deals with an independent risk factor for heart disease, but testing all of them at the same time increases the predictive value of your actual risk of a cardiovascular event.

In effect, doing all the tests, instead of just the standard lipid profile, increases the ability to predict your chances of having a heart attack or other circulatory problem from 50 percent to well over 90 percent.[55]

If you were investing in the stock market, would you be confident buying a stock with only a 50 percent likelihood of increasing in value? Or would you put your money on one whose chances of increasing in value were 90 percent? Isn't the same true when you are "investing" in your health? Don't settle for uncertainty just because some tests aren't covered by your insurance. Invest in your health. Find out where the potholes are in your wellness plan and then fix them!

GENETIC TESTING FOR ALZHEIMER'S AND CARDIOVASCULAR DISEASE

A blood or saliva test for the Apolipoprotein (ApoE) gene mutation can significantly help you understand your individualized risk for Alzheimer's disease. Ideally, you should have two normal copies of the ApoE3 gene (ApoE3 / E3). In those who develop Alzheimer's, the average age that symptoms begin is eighty-four, but only if they have two normal copies of the ApoE gene. If you have one ApoE3 gene and one mutated form (ApoE3 / E4), your risk of developing Alzheimer's can be increased from two to four times, and the average age that symptoms begin is seventy-five—nearly ten years younger than those with two normal copies of the ApoE gene. However, if you have two copies of the mutation (ApoE4 / E4), symptoms start, on average, at age sixty-eight,[56] and your risk increases dramatically—from 5 to 34 times greater. The average increased risk is eleven-fold or 1,100 percent![57]

That certainly can be a stressful thing to find out, but you need to know. By becoming aware, you can, at least recognize the risk and aggressively work on all the factors that influence Alzheimer's to reduce that risk as much as possible. It would be even worse to not know and find out fifteen or twenty years later—without being able to reduce the risk. And there *are* ways to reduce the risk of Alzheimer's. In fact, Alzheimer's is as much as 90 percent preventable if we know what the issues are and work on them aggressively well before the age of diagnosis.[58]

Genetic testing is still very misunderstood by many. Having a gene that is strongly associated with a given disease doesn't mean you will eventually develop that disease.

Dr. Carrie Hill, PhD has summarized key points that help us understand the relationship between the Apo E4 gene mutation and Alzheimer's:[59]

» At least 20 percent of those with Apo E4 do not develop Alzheimer's.

» 25 percent of individuals in the United States have at least one mutated copy.

» Half of those with Alzheimer's do not have the Apo E4 gene.

» Having one copy of ApoE4 carries the same risk as having one parent with Alzheimer's.

» Insurance plans don't typically cover Apo E gene testing.

Interestingly, the ApoE gene mutation test is part of the Hunter Heart Profile. It's included because the ApoE4 mutation increases the risk of cardiovascular disease by nearly 50 percent in men and doubles the risk in women.[60] This increase in risk is above and beyond all other health risk factors!

It is important to remember that whatever is good for the heart is also good for the brain. That's the beauty of focusing your treatment plan primarily on lifestyle and nutritional medicine approaches. When you improve one risk factor naturally, you often improve many others at the same time.

FACTOR V LEIDEN GENE MUTATION

Another gene test, the Factor V Leiden test, can determine if you have a tendency for blood clots, pulmonary embolisms (PE), or deep vein thrombosis (DVT).[61] For instance, having one copy of the mutation increases a person's risk of DVT five to sevenfold. Having two copies of this mutation increases the risk of DVT somewhere between 25 and 50 times! Women on birth control pills are three to four times more likely to get DVT or PE, but if they have the Factor V Leiden mutation and use birth control pills, they become 35 times more likely to develop these clotting disorders.[62] Is this something important to know? Absolutely. And there are very simple natural strategies you can follow to address those risk factors.

When the Hunter Heart Profile first became available as one of the most comprehensive advanced cardiac risk factor testing options, I chose to test myself right away. To my surprise, I tested positive for the Factor V Leiden genetic mutation and, therefore, for an increased risk of heart disease. From this lab report I learned that I was up to 800 percent more likely to experience a blood clot! This was great news to me. I'm serious! I was very grateful to discover this risk factor before it had a chance to damage my health. Because I love speaking on lifestyle medicine topics at medical conferences, corporate wellness programs, and to church groups, I spend a lot of time flying around the world. It just so happens that flying also increases the risk of blood clots forming. This is especially true if you have the Factor V Leiden gene mutation. With this new health awareness, I added a very important "page" to my personalized wellness plan. Specifically I now emphasize the following to lower my risk of getting blood clots:

1. At least 80 percent of my calories come from first-class foods. Of course, this was already part of my wellness plan, but it's especially important for me, because whole, unprocessed plant foods are loaded with nutrients and natural phytochemicals that prevent and even reverse blood clots before they significantly impair circulation of blood to critical organs.

2. Walk or participate in light to moderate exercises for at least ten minutes immediately after each meal.

3. Stay well hydrated by drinking at least one cup of water thirty minutes before, and two hours after, every meal. Inadequate water intake will thicken the blood and increase the risk of clotting.

4. Eat small amounts of nuts and seeds such as chia or flax. Take supplemental EPA and DHA oils with meals. This improves the absorption of many nutrients and greatly lowers any tendency to form blood clots.

5. Stay fit by participating in vigorous exercise three times per week.

6. Nutritionally bypass mutated genes! It is often possible to neutralize or stabilize the metabolic dysfunction arising from the mutation by supplying the specific nutrients that are lacking. For example, we can significantly lower the risk associated with the MTHFR mutation. This is done by optimizing intake of methyl B12, methyl folate, and other appropriate nutrients—strawberries, blueberries, and other berries, for example—that stabilize important metabolic and biochemical pathways in our cells.

There are other considerations as well but the above list is a great example of how each of us can develop a personalized wellness plan based on initiating a more in-depth health assessment.

LUKE'S STORY

When I first became acquainted with Luke he was 74 years old. He was proud of the fact that he had been a Navy seal back before they were called seals. They were called "frogmen," at that time, he told me. Luke was gifted with the physical strength and stamina required of this elite Navy group. His eyesight and hearing were so keen, his troops followed his lead unquestioningly, because he could see and hear things before anyone else. They felt safe following him.

But by the time I saw Luke, he'd had multiple heart attacks and strokes. His blood sugars were extremely high. His fasting blood sugar was running between 400 and 500. His hemoglobin A1C was at 13.4 percent. His homocysteine was 45. Luke was a metabolic nightmare. I could tell by looking in his eyes that he had lost hope.

We ran the stimulated C-peptide test on Luke, because he was injecting high doses of insulin multiple times daily. After the results came back, I said, "Luke, good news! Your pancreas is functioning fine. You should be able to make all the insulin you need if you start paying attention to the proper wellness strategies."

How do you think he reacted—this old former Navy frogman, who had once been among the most fit individuals anywhere? As soon as Luke learned that it was possible to reverse his condition, he embraced that possibility and began to implement the necessary strategies.

"I have shrapnel all up and down my back," he said. "The doctors can't take it out, because it's so close to my spinal cord. When I start walking, I seize up, because of that shrapnel. I seize up and can't move. But I've learned that if I adjust myself a little bit, before long my back unlocks, and I can walk a few minutes. I can't walk for twenty or thirty minutes at a time, but I can walk five minutes at a time. And I can do that five or six or eight times a day."

So Luke began working on reversing all the health problems he was facing. Before long he was able to completely quit taking his 200 units of insulin. He brought his blood sugars down to 100 before meals and 140 after meals. Hope had allowed Luke to bring his hemoglobin A1C down dramatically by more than half. By doing these things, he gave himself many more years of healthy life. No more depression, no more fatigue, all because he embraced his new-found awareness and then, like he had done so many times before as a Navy seal, aggressively addressed the underlying cause of his problem.

YOU CAN FIND A NEW DIRECTION IN LIFE

As we've emphasized throughout this book, it's important to recognize that your exposome—all those things in your life, your environment, the choices you make physically, emotionally, and attitudinally—can optimize your potential for epigenetic change.

> You can live a healthier, happier, richer, more joyful and fuller life. But it requires effort. It demands that you set limits. It will mean that you sometimes have to say No to things you really want to do, in order to say Yes to those things that will give you this richer, fuller life.

Setting limits doesn't mean limiting the joy in your life. It means dramatically and exponentially increasing your potential for joy. Show me someone who never sets limits for themselves, and I'll show you a depressed, damaged person. Show me someone who has set prudent, appropriate limits, and I'll show you a person who is happy and satisfied with life.

It begins with broad, comprehensive testing. Be willing to embrace the idea of assessment. Work with your healthcare team to develop a sound, solid program for personal health and wellness based on the results of the testing you have had. Follow the strategies. You can gain a new direction in life that will take you where you want to be.

CHAPTER SUMMARY

>> One of the most significant components of optimizing your health is to embrace the diagnosis—being willing to find out what is going on in your body.

>> Testing is indispensable to knowing the state of your body and what your health needs actually are.

>> The single most effective way to reduce your risk of heart disease is to correct insulin resistance.

>> Knowing the five stages of high blood sugars—and where you fit within them—allows you to take actions to improve, and possibly, reverse the condition.

» When it comes to testing, it's better to be safe than sorry.

» The glucose tolerance test is the most accurate and comprehensive test available for determining a predisposition for prediabetes or diabetes.

» You can do a modified glucose tolerance test on yourself using the "Pepsi®-Jelly Bean Challenge."

» The fasting insulin test measures the amount of insulin in the blood, before breakfast and after not eating since the previous evening.

» The C-Peptide test measures the health of the pancreas and how effectively it is producing insulin. It can help determine the likelihood of diabetes reversal even in someone currently taking insulin injections.

» The Comprehensive Metabolic Profile (CMP) is a broad spectrum test that reviews many body systems and how well they are functioning.

» The Hemoglobin A1C test (the "sticky blood sugar" test) is strongly influenced by how much your blood sugar spikes after meals and gives insight into your level of insulin resistance.

» Since the standard lipid (cholesterol) profile picks up less than half of the risk of having a heart attack, it's important to do advanced cardiac labs such as the Hunter Heart Profile.

» A blood or saliva test for the Apolipoprotein (ApoE) gene mutation helps you understand your risk for Alzheimer's disease and what you can start doing now to minimize that risk.

» Through proper effort and effectively setting limits, you can achieve your personal goals and live a healthier, happier life.

ENDNOTES

1 Proverbs 17:22, NKJV.

2 See Luke 14:28.

3 Weisberg, I, "The 1298A C Polymorphism in Methylenetetrahydrofolate Reductase (MTHFR): In Vitro Expression and Association With Homocysteine,"*Atherosclerosis*, 156 (2001), 409-415.

4 Wisotzkey, J, "MTHFR (C677T) Polymorphisms and Stage III Colon Cancer: Response to Therapy" *Molecular Diagnosis*, 4 (1999), 95-99.

5 Eddy, D, "Relationship of Insulin Resistance and Related Metabolic Variables to Coronary Artery Disease: A Mathematical Analysis," *Diabetes Care*, 32 (2009), 361-366.

6 Cowie, C, et al, "Full Accounting of Diabetes and Pre-Diabetes in the U.S. Population in 1988-1994 and 2005-2006," *Diabetes Care*, 32 (2009) 287–294.

7   Reaven, Gerald, "Insulin Resistance/Compensatory Hyperinsulinemia, Essential Hypertension, and Cardiovascular Disease," *The Journal of Clinical Endocrinology and Metabolism*, 88.6 (2003): 2399-2403.

8   Osterweil, Neil, "Elevated Insulin Increases Alzheimer's Disease Risk," MedPage Today, August 2005, accessed August 2012, http://www.medpagetoday.com/Neurology/ AlzheimersDisease/1506.

9   Barnard, R. James, "Prostate Cancer Prevention by Nutritional Means to Alleviate Metabolic Syndrome," *The American Journal of Clinical Nutrition*, 86.3, (2007): 889S-893S. Giovannucci, Edward, "Insulin and Colon Cancer," *Cancer Causes and Control*, 6.2 (1995): 164-179.

10 Reaven, Gerald, "Insulin Resistance/Compensatory Hyperinsulinemia, Essential Hypertension, and Cardiovascular Disease," *The Journal of Clinical Endocrinology and Metabolism*, 88.6 (2003): 2399-2403.

11 Simon, K, "Tests for Diagnosing Diabetes Mellitus. Glucose Tolerance Test Is Most Sensitive," *BMJ*, 309.6953 (1994), 537, 538.

12 National Library of Medicine, "Glucose Tolerance Test," Accessed July 2012, http://www.nlm.nih.gov/cgi/mesh/2011/MB_cgi?mode=&term=Glucose+Tolerance+Test.

13 American Diabetes Association, "Standards of Medical Care in Diabetes—2010," *Diabetes Care*, 33.1 (2010), 511-561.

14 National Diabetes Information Clearinghouse, "Diagnosis of Diabetes," National Institutes of Health. accessed July 2012, http://diabetes.niddk.nih.gov/dm/pubs/diagnosis/#what.

15 See Endnote 5.

16 Sciacqua, A, et al, "One-hour Postload Plasma Glucose Levels and Left Ventricular Mass in Hypertensive Patients," *Diabetes Care*, 34.6 (2011), 1406-1411.

17 Lamar, M. E., et al, "Jelly Beans as an Alternative to a Fifty-Gram Glucose Beverage for Gestational Diabetes Screening," *American Journal of Obstetrics and Gynecology*, 181.5 (1999), 1154-1157.

18 Cowie, Catherine, et. al., "Full Accounting of Diabetes and Pre-Diabetes in the U.S. Population in 1988-1994 and 2005-2006," *Diabetes Care*, 32.2 (2009), 287-294.

19 Lab Tests Online, "Insulin," accessed July 2012, http://labtestsonline.org/understanding/analytes/insulin/tab/test.

20 Mayo Clinic, "Type 2 Diabetes," accessed July 2012. http://www.mayoclinic.com/health/hyperinsulinemia/HQ00896.

21 Reaven, Gerald, "Insulin Resistance/Compensatory Hyperinculinemia, Essential Hypertension, and Cardiovascular Disease," *The Journal of Clinical Endocrinology and Metabolism*, 88.6 (2003), 2399-2403.

22 Despres, Jean-Pierre, et. al., "Hyperinsulinemia as an Independent Risk Factor for Ischemic Heart Disease," *The New England Journal of Medicine*, 334 (1996), 952-958.

23 Modan, Michaela, et al, "Hyperinsulinemia: A Link Between Hypertension Obesity and Glucose Intolerance," *Journal of Clinical Investigation*, 75 (1985), 809-817.

24 Barnard, R. James, "Prostate Cancer Prevention by Nutritional Means to Alleviate Metabolic Syndrome," *The American Journal of Clinical Nutrition*, 86.3 (2007), 889S-893S.

25 Giovannucci, Edward, "Insulin and Colon Cancer," *Cancer Causes and Control*, 6.2 (1995), 164-179.

26 Novosyadly, Ruslan and LeRoith, Derek, "Hyperinsulinemia and Type 2 Diabetes," *Cell Cycle*, 9.8 (2010), 1449, 1450.

27 Sakumoto, Tetsurou, et al, "Insulin Resistance/Hyperinsulinemia and Reproductive Disorders in Infertile Women," *Reproductive Medicine and Biology*, 9.4 (2010), 185.

28 Osterweil, Neil, "Elevated Insulin Increases Alzheimer's Disease Risk," MedPage Today, August 2005, accessed August 2012, http://www.medpagetoday.com/Neurology/Alzheimer'sDisease/1506.

29 Bohanon, Nancy, Family Practice Audio Digest, 1991, 1992.

30 Hyman, Mark, *The Blood Sugar Solution* (New York: Little, Brown and Company, 2012), 180.

31 Lab Tests Online, "C-Peptide," accessed July 2012, http://labtestsonline.org/understanding/analytes/c-peptide/tab/test.

32 WebMD, "Diabetes Health Center: C-peptide," accessed August 2012, http://diabetes.webmd.com/c-peptide.

33 Weinstock, Ruth and Zygmont, Steven, "Pancreatic Islet Function Tests," EndoText.org, January 2010, accessed August 2012, http://www.endotext.org/protocols/protocols5/protocols5.htm.

34 Personal interview, George Guthrie and Charles Zeno Marcell, American College of Lifestyle Medicine meeting, September 2006.

35 Swaminathan S., Fonseca,V.A., Alam M.G., Shah S.V., "The Role of Iron in Diabetes and Its Complications," *Diabetes Care*, 2007;30: 1926–1933.

36 Torti, Suzy V., Torti, Frank M., "Iron and Cancer: More Ore To Be Mined," *Nature Reviews Cancer*, 2013, 13, 5, 342.

37 Moore, E, "Cognitive Impairment and Vitamin B12: A Review," *Int Psychogeriatr*, April 24, 2012, (4):541-56. Seshadri, S, et al, "Plasma Homocysteine As a Risk Factor for Dementia and Alzheimer's Disease" *New England Journal of Medicine*, 2002 346: 476–483.

38 See Chapter 10, especially the section "Additional Tests for Toxicity" (pages xx to xx), for more information about homocysteine and its effects on the body.

39 Douaud, Gwenaelle; Refsum, Helga; de Jager, Celeste A.; Jacoby, Robin; Nichols, Thomas E.; Smith, Stephen M.; Smith, A. David; "Preventing Alzheimer's Disease-Related Gray Matter Atrophy by B-Vitamin Treatment," *Proc National Academy of Science*, USA, June 4, 2013, 110(23): 9523-9528.

40 Perna, Alessandra F., "Possible Mechanisms of Homocysteine Toxicity," *Kidney International* (2003) 63, S137–S140.

41 For more detailed information on the importance of Vitamin D and its effects on various aspects of health and wellness, see Chapter 4, "Sunlight, Vitamin D and Health," (pages 52-71).

42 Urashima, Mitsuyoshi, et al, "Randomized Trial of Vitamin D Supplementation to Prevent Seasonal Influenza A in Schoolchildren," *The American Journal of Clinical Nutrition*, 91.5 (2010):1255-1260. Ling, M., et al, "A Randomized Controlled Trial of Vitamin D3 Supplementation for the Prevention of Symptomatic Upper Respiratory Tract Infections," *Epidemiology and Infection*, 137.10 (2009):1396-1414.

43 Littlejohns, Thomas J.; Henley, William E.; Lang, Iain A.; et al., "Vitamin D and the Risk of Dementia and Alzheimer's Disease," *Neurology*, published online August 6, 2014.

44 Grassroots Health, "Disease Incidence Prevention by Serum 25(OH)D Level," March 2010, accessed September 2012. http://grassrootshealth.net/media/download/disease_incidence_prev_chart_032310.pdf. Garland, Cedric F., and Garland, Frank C., "Do Sunlight and Vitamin D Reduce the Likelihood of Colon Cancer?," *International Journal of Epidemiology*, 9.3(1980):227-231. Garland, Cedric F., et al, "The Role of Vitamin D in Cancer Prevention," *American Journal of Public Health*, 96.2 (2006):252-261. Holick, M. F., "Vitamin D and Sunlight: Strategies for Cancer Prevention and Other Health Benefits," *Clinical Journal of the American Society of Nephrology*, 3.5(2008):1548-1554.

45 Stratton, Irene, et al, "Association of Glycaemia with Macrovascular and Microvascular Complications of Type 2 Diabetes (UKPDS 35): Prospective Observational Study," *BMJ*, 321.7258 (2000): 405-412.

46 Ridker, P., et al., "Rosuvastatin to Prevent Vascular Events in Men and Women With Elevated C-Reactive Protein," *New England Journal of Medicine*, 2008; 359: 2195-2207.

47 Lanman, R. B.; Wolfert, R. L.; Fleming, J. K.; et al., "Lipoprotein-Associated Phospholipase A2: Review and Recommendation of a Clinical Cut Point for Adults," *Prev Cardiol*, 2005;9(3): 138-143.

48 Ballantyne, C. M.; Hoogeveen, R. C.; Bang, H.; et al., "Lipoprotein-Associated Phospholipase A2, High-Sensitivity C-Reactive Protein, and Risk for Incident Ischemic Stroke in Middle-Aged Men and Women in the Atherosclerosis Risk in Communities (ARIC) Study," *Arch Intern Med*, November 28, 2005, 165(21):2479-2484.

49 Mannheim, D., "Enhanced Expression of Lp-PLA and Mannheim Lysophosphatidylcholine in Symptomatic Carotid Atherosclerotic Plaques," *Stroke*. 2008;39:1448-1455.

50 Ridker, P., "Proposed Cardiovascular Risk Assessment Algorithm Using High-Sensitivity C-Reactive Protein and Lipid Screening," *Clinical Chemistry*, January 2001, vol. 47, o. 1; 28-30.

51 Hall, J. L., "Lipoprotein(a) As a Potential Causal Genetic Risk Factor of Cardiovascular Disease: A Rationale for Increased Efforts to Understand Its P\athophysiology and Develop Targeted Therapies," *Journal of the American College of Cardiology*, August 212, 2012, 60(8):716-721.

52 "Optimizing Patient Cardiovascular Care with the Hunter Heart Profile," a 2014 presentation by Paul Ziajka, M.D., Ph.D., Director of The Florida Lipid Institute; Diplomat of the American Board of Clinical Lipidology; President of the South East Lipid Association.

53 See Endnote 50.

54 Tian L., et al. "Characteristics of High-Density Lipoprotein Subclasses Distribution for Subjects With Desirable Total Cholesterol Levels." *Lipids in Health and Disease*, 2011; 10: 64-72.

55 See Endnote 50.

56 Corder, E, "Gene Dose of Apolipoprotein E Type 4 Allele and the Risk of Alzheimer's Disease in Late Onset Families," *Science*, August 13, 1993, vol. 261, no. 5123, pp. 921-923.

57 Henrichs, I.; Froesch, D.; Wolf, A. S.; Teller, W. M.; "Impact of Apolipoprotein E on Alzheimer's Disease," *Current Alzheimer Research*, (2013) 10 (8): 809–817. http://www.netplaces.com/alzheimers/understanding-alzheimers-risks/genetic-risks-for-alzheimers.htm.

58 See Endnote 50.

59 See http://www.netplaces.com/alzheimers/understanding-alzheimers-risks/genetic-risks-for-alzheimers.htm.

60 Stengard, J. H.; Weiss, K. M.; Sing, C. F.; "An Ecological Study of Association Between Coronary Heart Disease Mortality Rates in Men and the Relative Frequencies of Common Allelic Variations in the Gene Coding for Apolipoprotein E," *Human Genetics*, 1998; 103:234–241. Eichner , J. E.; Kuller, L. H.; Orchard, T. J.; et al.; "Relation of Apolipoprotein E Phenotype to Myocardial Infarction and Mortality from Coronary Artery Disease, *American Journal of Cardiology*, 1993, 71:160–165. Lehtinen, S.; Lehtimaki, T.; Sisto, T.; et al.; "Apolipoprotein E Polymorphism, Serum Lipids, Myocardial Infarction, and Severity of Angiography Verified Coronary Artery Disease in Men and Women," *Atherosclerosis*, 1995; 114:83–91.

61 Ornstein, D., Cardiology Patient Page—Factor V Leiden, *Circulation*, 2003; 107: e94-e97.

62 See Endnote 59.

CREATING A FIRST-CLASS NUTRITIONAL PLAN FOR OPTIMAL HEALTH

[Adapted from Chapter 13 of *Goodbye Diabetes*]

CURRENT NUTRITIONAL RESEARCH REGULARLY provides us with important information about the nutrients our bodies need. Dietary studies continue to point to the kinds of foods that promote health and help protect us from illness and disease. Yet this valuable information becomes beneficial only when (and *if*) we put it into practice. An important part of your over-all wellness strategy is to make informed, healthful choices regarding the foods you eat. This appendix will help you establish an action plan to for incorporating a first-class diet into your lifestyle.

Eating a healthful, nutrient-dense diet is actually pretty simple. Foods can be divided into three categories: first-class, second-class, and third-class. Your health is great affected by which class of foods you primarily eat. The first step in creating a first-class nutritional plan for optimal health is to start eating more first-class foods.

FIRST-CLASS FOODS

If you want first-class health, you need to eat first-class foods. First-class foods include vegetables, beans/legumes, fruits, unrefined whole grains, nuts, and seeds. These plant-based foods are packed with powerful nutrients, fiber, antioxidants, phytochemicals, vitamins, and minerals. They also contain healthful carbohydrates, healthful proteins, and healthful fats.

Not only do first-class foods provide you with optimal energy and help you feel your best, but they also protect you against diabetes, heart disease, cancer, and a host of other diseases.[1][2][3][4] I recommend that you eat at least 80 to 90 percent of your calories from first-class foods. Let's take a closer look at what these foods are, starting with those most dense in nutrients—green leafy vegetables.

FIRST-CLASS FOODS[5]		
Food	**Examples**	**Benefits**
Green Leafy Vegetables[6,7]	Romain lettuce, spinach, broccoli, kale, collards, turnip greens, mustard greens, cabbage, arugula, Swiss chard, bok choy	The most nutrient-dense of all plant foods, green leafy veggies are rich in dietary fiber, calcium, magnesium, minerals, vitamins, and other phytonutrients.
Green Vegetables	Green beans, asparagus, cucumbers, zucchini, green bell peppers, Brussels sprouts, artichokes, celery, sprouts	Green vegetables provide an abundant amount of phytonutrients for optimal health.
Colorful Vegetables	Carrots, tomatoes, purple cabbage, bell peppers, eggplant, squash, beets, cauliflower, onions, turnips, garlic, leeks	The colorful pigments of these vegetables are rich in special forms of flavornoids and antioxidants.
Beans/Legumes	Pinto beans, black beans, kidney beans, lentils, garbanzos/chick peas, lima beans, white beans, black-eyed peas, soybeans, fava beans, mung beans	Beans are rich in fiber, protein, carbohydrates, and other nutrients. Beans help control and stabilize blood sugars.
Starchy Vegetables	Sweet potatoes, yams, baked potatoes, corn, peas	Rich sources of carbohydrates, fiber, and other nutrients, these starchy vegetables need to be balanced with healthful proteins and fats.

FIRST-CLASS FOODS[5]		
Food	Examples	Benefits
Fresh Fruits	Apples, oranges, tangerines, grapefruits, pears, grapes, berries, bananas, melons, apricots, cherries, coconuts, kiwis, lemons, limes, nectarines, peaches, plums, strawberries	Good sources of energy with fiber, natural antioxidants, and vitamins, these fruits need to be balanced with healthful proteins and fats.
Whole, Unrefined Grains	Barley, oatmeal, oat groats, quinoa, brown rice, wild rice, Kamut®, bulgar (cracked wheat), buckwheat, millet, amaranth, spelt	Whole grains provide fiber and other nutrients missing in refined carbohydrates. These starches need to be balanced with healthful proteins and fats.
Raw Nuts and Seeds	Walnuts, almonds, pecans, cashews, hazelnuts, macadamia nuts, pistachios, pine nuts, pumpkin seeds, sesame seeds, flax seeds, chia seeds, poppy seeds, sunflower seeds, old-fashioned peanut butter, almond butter, sunflower butter	Nuts and seeds are good sources of heart-healthy fats, protein, and other nutrients. Because of their high fat content, they should be used moderately.
Whole-Food Fats	Whole olives, whole avocados, whole coconuts, nuts, seeds	Good sources of healthful fat and other nutrients, but high in calories. Should be used moderately.
First-Class Beverages: Water, Fresh-pressed Vegetable Juices	A wide variety of vegetables can be included in these juices. Minimal fruit can be added to enhance flavor without spiking blood sugars.	Water is your beverage of choice. Be sure to stay well hydrated by drinking plenty of water throughout the day. Fresh-pressed vegetable juices are high in nutrients and phytochemicals.

SECOND-CLASS FOODS

Second-class foods are not nearly as nutrient-rich as first-class foods. That's why I recommend that only a small percentage of your calories come from these foods. Not all second-class foods are created equal. I have attempted to list them in order of decreasing nutritional value. Depending on your current health status and dietary preferences, you may want to avoid some second-class foods altogether.

SECOND-CLASS FOODS		
Food	**Example**	**Benefits/Dangers**
Processed Whole Grains	Whole-wheat or whole-grain bread or pasta (or other whole-wheat flour products), whole-grain cereal, couscous	These refined whole-grain foods are more healthful than foods made with white flour. However, they are still processed foods and generally spike blood sugars more than unrefined whole grains.
Processed Fruits or Vegetables (with added sugar, salt, or fat)	Applesauce, canned fruits with added sugar, dried fruits with added sugar, canned and salted vegetables	Processed foods are not as healthful as fresh fruits and can raise blood sugars more dramatically. Processed vegetables lose many of their nutrients and can be high in sodium and fat.
Milk Alternatives	Soy milk, almond and other nut milks	These milk-replacement products are more healthful alternatives to real milk. They can be used in cereal, smoothies, etc. Be sure to choose unsweetened varieties.
Meat Substitutes	Soy burgers, veggie burgers, soy hot dogs, textured vegetable protein	Imitation meats are lower in saturated fat and cholesterol than real meats. However, it's important to be selective and read the labels! These products are processed foods and should be used moderately.
Organic, Fat-free Dairy and Free-range Eggs	Organic, fat-free milk, yogurt, and cottage cheese	These foods are lower in saturated fat and cholesterol than regular dairy products. Organic forms are safer to eat. However, dairy is not an optimal food for humans. It it's consumed, it should be on a limited basis. Free-range eggs are high in saturated fat and cholesterol, but are safer to eat than regular eggs. Using only egg whites removes the fat and cholesterol.
Cold-water Fish	Mackerel, trout, herring, water-packed tuna, and salmon	These fish are high in omega-3 fatty acids. However, many fish contain mercury and other dangerous toxins.[8] A better option is to take a DHA/EPA-rich, microalgae supplement or an omega-rich purified fish oil. Flax seeds and walnuts also contain some omega-3 fatty acids. Pregnant and lactating women are especially encouraged to limit fish intake.

SECOND-CLASS FOODS		
Food	Example	Benefits/Dangers
White Meat	Chicken and turkey	White meat contains less saturated fat than red meat, but it contains the same amount of cholesterol. If you choose to eat these meats, it's best to use organic products to avoid contamination associated with hormones, antibiotics, etc. [9]
Virgin Oils (use sparingly)	Extra virgin, cold-pressed olive oil, coconut oil, flax seed oil, hemp seed oil, EFA oil blends	It's best to get fats from whole plant sources such as olives, avocados, coconuts, nuts, and seeds. However, if you choose to use oil, use extra virgin, cold-pressed forms for baking and try an essential oil blend for salad dressings.
Second-class Beverages: Fruit Juices	100% fruit juice	Fruit juice contains vitamins and minerals. However, even 100%, all-natural juice can spike blood sugars and contribute to weight gain. It's better to eat whole fruit than to drink fruit juice. Use juices sparingly and only on special occasions.

My personal goal is to eat a balanced variety of mostly first-class foods. I also incorporate into my diet some second-class foods such as whole-wheat bread and pasta, small amounts of virgin oils, non-dairy milks, meat substitutes, and egg whites. I avoid dairy as much as possible. I do not eat fish or meat. My diet isn't perfect, but I strive to make healthful choices. However, I recognize that different people have different dietary habits. My goal is not to make you eat exactly like I do, but to encourage you to move toward optimal health.

If you are regularly eating third-class foods, such as processed or red meats, it would be a step in the right direction to switch to second-class organic chicken and have it only a few times a week, combined with first-class foods. While I personally believe that moving toward a whole-food, total vegetarian diet is the best option for preventing and reversing disease, I understand that not everyone will choose to completely avoid meat and animal products. If you fall into this category, I want to give you more healthful options that will work for you.

If you're a vegetarian (you don't eat meat, fish, or poultry) or a vegan (you don't eat meat, fish, poultry, dairy, or eggs), then the animal products listed in the second-class foods obviously aren't the best choices for you. You will benefit greatly from focusing primarily on first-class foods, eating vegetarian second-class foods sparingly, and avoiding vegetarian third-class foods such as refined grains and sweets. Remember, although a vegetarian diet can be extremely healthful and beneficial, there are many unhealthful foods (and unhealthy people) who are vegetarian. Dr. Joel Fuhrman encourages his patients to be "nutritarians" by eating a nutrient-rich diet.[10] If you're a vegetarian, make sure you're a nutritarian too!

THIRD-CLASS FOODS

There's no getting around it—third-class foods are simply bad for your health. These foods have been shown to promote inflammation, raise triglycerides and cholesterol, increase insulin resistance, and significantly raise your risk for disease. Ideally, these foods should be completely avoided, but if included in your diet, it should be on a *very* limited basis.

THIRD-CLASS FOODS		
Food	Example	Benefits/Dangers
Refined Grains	White bread (or any bread that doesn't say, "100% whole grain"), white flour, white rice, white pasta, etc.	Refined grains promote inflammation, raise triglycerides, and spike blood sugars. They are also low in nutrients.
Refined Sweets	Cakes, pies, pastries, cookies, candy, sodas, artificially sweetened candy and desserts	Refined sweets have a worse impact on inflammation, triglycerides, and blood sugars than do even refined grains. Most artificially sweetened foods contain damaging, disease-promoting chemicals.
Cheese/Dairy	Cheese, yogurt, cottage cheese, sour cream	These foods are full of saturated fat and cholesterol.
Regular Oils	Non-virgin vegetable oils, shortening, lard	Major sources of empty calories. Lard and shortening contain high amounts of either saturated or hydrogenated fat.

THIRD-CLASS FOODS		
Food	**Example**	**Benefits/Dangers**
Processed, Packaged Foods	Margarines, baking mixes, frozen entrees and waffles, fast food, canned soup, potato chips, cookies, microwave popcorn, and many other snack foods	Besides the high sodium, fat, and sugar often found in these products, they can also be a source of trans fat. These harmful fats increase the risk of heart disease, diabetes, and cancer even more than do saturated fats. Read the ingredients and avoid products that contain hydrogenated or partially hydrogenated oils.
Deep-fried Foods, Fast Food, and Restaurant-fried Foods	French fries, onion rings, chicken nuggets, fried chicken, fried fish, egg rolls, samosas	These foods are notorious for their high fat, sugar, and sodium content. Deep-fried animal products are also laden with saturated fat and cholesterol.
Red Meat	Beef, lamb, pork, veal	Very high in saturated fat and cholesterol. Known to significantly increase risk of diabetes, heart disease, cancer and other diseases.[13, 14]
Processed Meats	Hot dogs, hamburgers, salami, sausage, SPAM®, jerky, ground beef	Processed meats are even worse than red meats. They dramatically increase risk of many diseases, including diabetes, cancer, and heart disease.
Third-class Beverages: Sodas, Natural and Artificially Sweetened Beverages, and Caffeinated Beverages	Sodas. fruit drinks, sports drinks, energy drinks, coffee, caffeinated tea, artificially sweetened beverages	These beverages are loaded with sugar and calories, but are depleted in nutrients. Avoid these over-stimulating beverages. Low- or zero-calorie, artificially sweetened beverages contain unhealthful chemicals and should be completed avoided.

QUALITY AND QUANTITY

You now have a basic understanding of what an optimal diet consists of. You know the healthful foods to eat and the harmful foods to avoid. In short, you have learned about the *quality* of foods. First-class foods are the best, and third-class foods are the worst. Choosing high-quality, first-class foods will start you on your path to better health. But in addition to choosing the best *quality* of foods, you also need to eat the right quantity of food. This is where meal balancing comes in.

MEAL BALANCING

Optimal health requires that you not only eat the right *quality* of foods, but that you also eat the right *quantity* of those foods. That is what meal balancing is all about. To balance your meals, you need to eat the right amounts of healthful proteins, carbohydrates, and fats that come from first-class foods. The key is that all three nutrients—proteins, carbohydrates, and fats—should be present at each meal.

I encourage my patients to eat three meals a day, including a light supper early in the evening. I find this especially helpful for people who are trying to lose weight or improve sleep. I also advise patients to avoid snacking and to follow a consistent mealtime schedule.

BALANCING HEALTHFUL PROTEINS

Every meal should include a source of healthful proteins. When healthful proteins are added to carbohydrate-rich foods, they help slow down sugar absorption and balance blood sugar levels. First-class, protein-rich foods such as beans, lentils, nuts, and seeds should be added to meals containing carbohydrates. Second-class protein foods, such as meat substitutes, eggs, dairy, and white meats do not control blood sugars nearly as well as first-class protein foods even though they have similar amount of protein. Many of my patients have found that eating beans or lentils with a meal helps to control blood sugars—not just for that meal, but for up to the next three meals. Aim for two servings of healthful protein per meal—or a total of six servings per day (more about serving sizes later).

BALANCING HEALTHFUL CARBOHYDRATES

Every meal should include healthful carbs. Carbohydrate-rich foods such as whole grains, starchy vegetables, and fruits contain a variety of powerful nutrients. However, carbohydrates are made up of glucose (sugar) molecules that can very easily affect blood sugars. Not all carbs are created equal. First-class carbs are better for blood sugars than are second-class carbs, which are better than third-class carbs. Because there are so many types of carbohydrate foods, it is often a challenge to control carb portions—and in turn, to control blood sugars. Carbohydrate foods include:

» grains (rice, bread, pasta, noodles, cereal, etc.)

» starchy vegetables (potatoes, sweet potatoes, corn, etc.)

» sugars (white sugar, cakes, cookies, candy, sodas, etc.)

» non-starchy vegetables

» legumes (beans, peas, lentils)

CARB COUNTING

Several methods are available to help you keep track of your carbohydrate intake. One of the most common methods is carb counting. This involves counting the number of carbohydrate servings consumed in each meal and limiting them to healthful amounts that will help you control your weight and blood sugar levels.

Because not all carbs are created equal, they aren't all counted the same. Some foods that contain carbohydrates should be counted, while others don't need to be. I recommend keeping track of (1) your starchy carbohydrate intake, and (2) your fruit intake.

COUNTING STARCHY CARBS

Depending on your current health status, I recommend eating one to three servings of starchy carbohydrates (grains or starchy vegetables) per meal. One serving of carbohydrates equals fifteen grams, so one to three servings would be fifteen to forty-five grams of carbohydrates per meal. Here are some examples of one serving (fifteen grams) of carbohydrates:

» 1 slice whole wheat bread

» ½ cup oatmeal

» ⅓ cup rice or pasta

» 1 six-inch tortilla

» ¼ baked potato (3 ounces)

» ½ cup corn, sweet potatoes, winter squash, or mashed or boiled potatoes

If you are diabetic or prediabetic, overweight, or struggling with high triglycerides, the lower end of this 1-to-3-serving range is ideal for you. Cutting out excess starchy carbs will help you lose weight and lower your blood sugars and triglycerides. Be sure to check your blood sugar levels frequently to monitor how carbohydrates affect you. If your after-meal sugar levels are spiking after eating three servings per meal, you need to cut back. The amount of carbs you can handle may increase somewhat once your health has stabilized.

Remember that the whole, unrefined grains mentioned in the first-class foods section (oatmeal, barley, quinoa, wild rice, etc.) are better for blood sugar control than second-class processed whole grains (processed brown rice, whole grain bread or pasta, and other whole wheat flour products). Third-class refined grains (white rice, white bread, white pasta, etc.) and refined sweets (cookies, pastries, etc.) are the worst for blood sugar control. These carbs should be greatly minimized or avoided completely.

COUNTING FRUIT

In addition to starchy carbs, you also need to count your fruit carbs. I recommend eating 3 to 5 servings of fruit per day (roughly 1 to 2 servings per meal). Examples of a single serving of fruit (15 grams of carbs) include:

»   1 small fresh fruit (4 ounces)

»   ½ cup canned fruit (in its own juice)

»   ¼ cup dried fruit (2 tablespoons)

»   17 small grapes (3 ounces)

»   1 cup melon or berries

If you eat half a cup of oatmeal with apple slices for breakfast, this could equate to one serving of starchy carb and one serving of fruit. For another starchy carb serving, you could add a slice of whole wheat toast. To add healthful protein to your meal, you could spread peanut butter on your toast.

Remember, there are many carbohydrate foods. Servings add up quickly. Anytime you eat starches, grain products, fruits, sweetened beverages, sweets, or desserts, they all need to be counted toward your carbohydrate limits. Individual needs vary, depending on caloric needs and blood sugar control.

Some people may need to stay in the lower end of these ranges, while others may stay closer to the high end. Those who are more metabolically active may be able to exceed these recommended limits. It's crucial to monitor your blood sugars to determine how different amounts of various carbs affect you.

CARBS THAT DON'T COUNT (THE SAME WAY)

Beans and legumes are high in carbohydrates. However, they are also high in fiber and protein, and they have a remarkable ability to help stabilize blood sugars. For this reason, their carbohydrate content doesn't have to be included in the usual carbohydrate count. Beans and legumes need only to be counted as protein servings. Beans and legumes that contain added sugar (such as baked beans) are an exception to this rule.

Non-starchy vegetables are high in fiber and low in carbohydrates. These veggies don't need to be counted, but can be eaten liberally. Try to eat at least six servings of non-starchy veggies a day. If you're still hungry at the end of your meal, you can reach for more veggies—like kale, broccoli, greens, cabbage, cauliflower, cucumbers, or tomatoes. The list goes on and on! I encourage you to maximize your non-starchy vegetable intake as much as possible.

BALANCING HEALTHFUL FATS

Healthful fats slow digestion, which slows the release of sugar into the bloodstream. The healthful fats contained in olives, avocados, nuts, and seeds should be combined with healthful carbohydrates and proteins for optimal blood sugar control. Aim for 15 to 25 percent of your total calories to come from fat. This amount will vary by individual, but a person on a 1,500-calorie diet would consume approximately 25 to 42 grams of fat per day—or 8 to 14 grams of fat per meal. In the breakfast example above, you might add almonds or ground flax seed to your oatmeal.

FIBER—THE SECRET WEAPON

Fiber is key to blood sugar control. The fiber contained in plant foods helps naturally slow the absorption of sugar into the bloodstream. You goal should be to eat at least 35 to 50 grams of fiber every day. Healthful proteins such as beans and legumes, healthful carbs such as whole grains and fruit, and healthful fats such as nuts and seeds—all contain this secret weapon. That's why choosing first-class foods is an important strategy for blood sugar control.

The following table gives you a basic idea of how to balance your meals for optimal health.

A DAY IN THE LIFE OF A FIRST-CLASS FOODIE

Food	Servings Per Day/Meal	Serving Size
Non-Starchy Vegetables (including green leafy and colored non-starchy vegetables)	6 or more servings (usually split between lunch and dinner)	1 cup raw or 1/2 cup cooked or chopped
Healthful Carbohydrates (whole-grain starches, starchy vegetables, fruits)	1–3 servings per meal (15–45 grams of carbohydrate). Carbohydrate needs can vary and may be increased for people who are more metabolically active.	1 serving = 15 grams of carbohydrate 1 slice whole-grain bread 1/2 cup cooked whole-grain cereal 1/2 cup corn, squash, or potato 1/3 cup brown rice
Healthful Carbohydrates (fruit)	1–2 servings per meal (3–5 servings per day.)	1 piece small fruit (apple, orange, pear, etc.), 1/2 banana, or 1/2 cup chopped fruit
Healthful Proteins	2 servings per meal (6 servings per day)	1 serving = 7 grams protein 1/2 cup beans or lentils 1 ounce nuts or 2 tablespoons nut butter 1/2 cup (4 ounces) tofu
Healthful Fats	No more than 15–25% of your total calories should come from fat. 2–3 servings per meal (25–42 grams per day on 1,500 calories) 3–4 servings per meal (33–55 grams per day on 2,000 calories)	1 serving = 5 grams fat 1/8 large avocado, 1 teaspoon oil, 7 large olives, 1/4 ounce nuts, 2 teaspoons old-fashioned peanut or almond butter, 1 teaspoon extra virgin oil.

THE PLATE METHOD

The plate method can help you visualize these concepts in a more practical way by dividing your plate into three sections. Fill half your plate with non-starchy vegetables, a fourth of your plate with healthful proteins, and a fourth of your plate with healthful carbohydrates (starches and/or whole-grain carbohydrates). Fruit, also a carbohydrate, can be reserved as a healthful dessert option. Healthful fats and nuts can be incorporated to any part of your plate as appropriate.

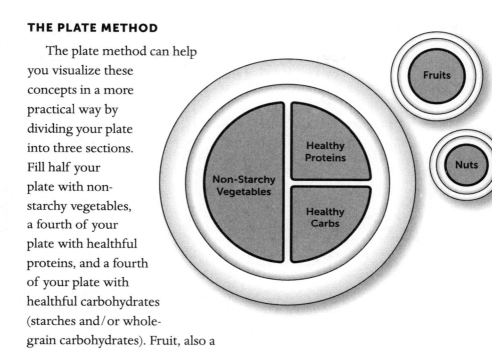

PUTTING IT ALL TOGTHER

You now have several tools to help you create a first-class nutritional plan for optimal health.

» First, choose first-class, nutrient-dense foods.

» Second, balance healthful carbs, proteins, and fats in appropriate portions and serving sizes.

» Third, use the plate method to fill your plate.

These three steps—together with the nutritional information you now have—will make you a "first-class foodie" and move you significantly further along the path to reaching your goal of optimal health and wellness.

ENDNOTES

1 Craig, W. J. and Mangels, A. R., "Position of the American Dietetic Association: Vegetarian Diets," *Journal of the American Dietetic Association,* 109.7 (2009): 1266-1282.

2 Craig, W. J., "Nutrition Concerns and Health Effects of Vegetarian Diets," *Nutrition in Clinical Practice,* 25.6 (2010): 613-620.

3 Craig, W. J., "Health Effects of Vegan Diets," *The American Journal of Clinical Nutrition,* 89.5 (2009): 1627S-1633S.

4 Hung, H. C., et al., "Fruit and Vegetable Intake and Risk of Major Chronic Disease," *Journal of the National Cancer Institute,* 96.21 (2004); 1577-1584.

5 Fuhrman, Joel, *Eat To Live* (New York, NY): Little, Brown and Company, (2011): 118-120.

6 American Institute for Cancer Research, "Foods That Fight Cancer: Dark Green Leafy Vegetables," accessed July 2012, http://preventcancer.aicr.org/site/PageServer?pagename=foodsthatfightcancer_leafy_vegetables.

7 Joshipura, K. J., et al., "The Effect of Fruit and Vegetable Intake on Risk for Coronary Heart Disease," *Annals of Internal Medicine,* 134.12 (2001): 1106-1114.

8 Manning, Anita, "If You Eat a Lot of Fish, You May Run Health Risk," *USA Today,* November 2002, accessed July 2012, http://www.usatoday.com/news/health/2002-11-04-fish-1acover_x.htm.

9 Hoffman, Matthew, "Safer Food For a Healthier You," Webmd.com, accessed July 2012, http://www.webmd.com/diet/features/safer-food-healthier-you.

10 Fuhrman, Joel, *Eat To Live* (New York, NY): Little, Brown and Company, (2011): 165.

11 Masters, Rachel, C., et al., "Whole and Refined Grain Intakes Are Related to Inflammatory Protein Concentrations in Human Plasma," *The Journal of Nutrition,* 140.3 (2010)): 587-594.

12 Liu, Simin, "Intake of Refined Carbohydrates and Whole Grain Foods in Relation to Risk of Type 2 Diabetes Mellitus and Coronary Heart Disease," *Journal of the American College of Nutrition,* 21.4 (2002): 298-306.

13 Pan, An, et al., "Red Meat Consumption and Mortality: Results from Two Prospective Cohort Studies," *Archives of Internal Medicine,* 172.7 (2012): 555-563.

14 Pan, An, et al., "Red Meat Consumption and Risk of Type 2 Diabetes: Three Cohorts of U.S. Adults and an Updated Meta-Analysis," *The American Journal of Clinical Nutrition,* August 2011, accessed July 2012, http://www.ajcn.org/content/early/2011/08/10/ajcn.111.018978.abstract.

15 See Endnote 14.

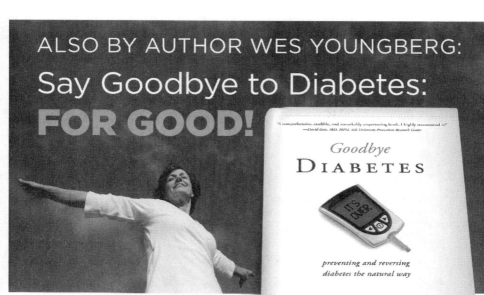
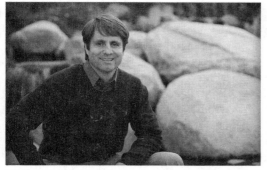

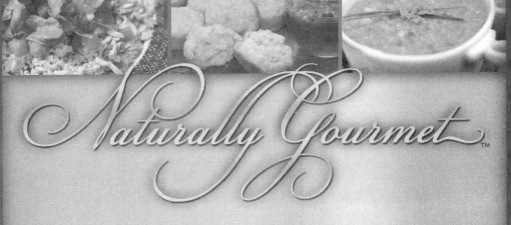

Naturally Gourmet™

Karen Houghton, RN, BSN, shares simple, plant-based recipes that are healthy & delicious!

If you're looking for a way to eat more healthfully without sacrificing flavor, *Naturally Gourmet*™ is a must for your kitchen and television screen! The cookbook features more than 100 beautifully photographed, plant-based recipes that are not only mouthwateringly good, but easy to prepare. The DVD series includes 14 enjoyable thirty-minute programs featuring host **Karen Houghton,** with special guest **Dr. Wes Youngberg.** You'll discover healthy tips for battling heart disease, diabetes, obesity and more!

Visit **www.NaturallyGourmet.com** or call **760-723-8082** to order your copies today!